....
Epidemiology of Pediatric Sports Injuries

Medicine and Sport Science

Vol. 49

Series Editors

J. Borms   *Brussels*
M. Hebbelinck   *Brussels*
A.P. Hills   *Brisbane*

KARGER

Epidemiology of Pediatric Sports Injuries

Team Sports

Volume Editors

Nicola Maffulli   *Stoke on Trent*
Dennis J. Caine   *Bellingham, Wash.*

1 figure and 40 tables, 2005

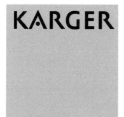

KARGER

Basel · Freiburg · Paris · London · New York ·
Bangalore · Bangkok · Singapore · Tokyo · Sydney

Medicine and Sport Science

Founder and Editor from 1969 to 1984: E. Jokl†, Lexington, Ky.

....

Nicola Maffulli, MD, MS, PhD, FRCS (Orth)

Department of Trauma and Orthopedic Surgery
Keele University School of Medicine
Stoke on Trent ST4 7QB
England

Dennis J. Caine, PhD

Department of Physical Education, Health and Recreation
Western Washington University
Bellingham, WA 98225-9067, USA

Library of Congress Cataloging-in-Publication Data

Epidemiology of pediatric sports injuries.
   v. ; cm. – (Medicine and sport science ; v. 48-)
  Includes bibliographical references and index.
  Contents: [1] Individual sports / volume editors, Dennis J.
Caine, Nicola Maffulli.
  ISBN 3-8055-7868-7 (v. 1 : hard cover : alk. paper)
  1. Pediatric sports medicine. 2. Sports injuries in children.
  I. Caine, Dennis John, 1949-   . II. Maffulli, Nicola. III.
Series.
  [DNLM: 1. Athletic Injuries–epidemiology–Adolescent. 2.
Athletic
  Injuries–epidemiology–Child. 3. Sports Medicine–Adolescent.
  4. Sports Medicine–Child.   W1 ME649Q v.48-49 2005 / QT 261
  E638 2005]
  RC1218.C45E65 2005
  617.1′027′083–dc22

    2004024872

Bibliographic Indices. This publication is listed in bibliographic services, including Current Contents® and Index Medicus.

Drug Dosage. The authors and the publisher have exerted every effort to ensure that drug selection and dosage set forth in this text are in accord with current recommendations and practice at the time of publication. However, in view of ongoing research, changes in government regulations, and the constant flow of information relating to drug therapy and drug reactions, the reader is urged to check the package insert for each drug for any change in indications and dosage and for added warnings and precautions. This is particularly important when the recommended agent is a new and/or infrequently employed drug.

© Copyright 2005 by S. Karger AG, P.O. Box, CH–4009 Basel (Switzerland)
www.karger.com
Printed in Switzerland on acid-free paper by Reinhardt Druck, Basel
ISSN 0254–5020
ISBN 3–8055–7869–5

Contents

Maffulli N, Caine DJ (eds): Epidemiology of Pediatric Sports Injuries: Team Sports.
Med Sport Sci. Basel, Karger, 2005, vol 49, pp 1–8

....

The Epidemiology of Children's Team Sports Injuries

An Important Area of Medicine and Sport Science Research

Nicola Maffulli[a], *Dennis Caine*[b]

[a]Keele University School of Medicine, University Hospital of North Staffordshire
and Hartshill Orthopedic Surgical Unit, Stoke on Trent, Staffordshire, England;
[b]Department of Physical Education, Health and Recreation, Western Washington
University, Bellingham, Wash., USA

Introduction

Participation in children's and youth sports is increasingly popular and widespread in Western culture. Many of these youngsters initiate year-round training and specialization in their sports at a very early age. This is probably due to the 'catch them young' philosophy, and to the belief that, to achieve international standing in later sporting life, intensive training should be started before puberty [1]. It is not uncommon, for example, for preteens to train 20 or more hours each week at regional training centers in tennis or gymnastics, to compete in triathlons, or for youngsters as young as 6–8 years of age to play organized hockey or soccer and travel with select teams to other towns and communities to compete against other teams of similar caliber.

The first volume of our work on the epidemiology of sports injuries in children dealt with individual sports. Organized team sport has become a feature of sports participation in Western children and adolescents, and, especially at school level, more than one team sport may well be practiced on a regular basis. This second volume concentrates on team sports. In this introductory article, we shall reiterate and expand on the general concepts on sports participation in young athletes already outlined in the first volume, and shall highlight some of the peculiarities of participation in team sports.

Peculiarities of Participation in Team Sports

In team sports one cannot consider the athletes in and by themselves, but only as part of a team. Hence, individuality may be lost. Also, the features of team sport are such that one does not compete against time, or to set a record expressed in weight, time, distance or height, but 'to win', and that victory is not necessarily dependent on the absolute number of points scored. Although some team sports are, theoretically, noncontact, in reality most of them involve some elements of contact with other players, and this influences the features of the injuries seen. The psychology of team-sport participants is also different: participants in team sports must be able to interact with the other members of the team, need to be able to sacrifice their skills and wishes for the greater good of the team, and may have to learn to renege on the *prima donna* role that they may feel they were born to play [2]. Finally, as many team sports involve the ability to be in the right place at the right time, the motor skills required are varied, and may well be different from what is required for individual sports.

Injury and Growth

Engaging in sports activities at a young age has numerous health benefits but also involves risk of injury. Indeed, the young athlete may be particularly vulnerable to sport injury due to the physical and physiological processes of growth. Injury risk factors unique to the growing athlete include: susceptibility to growth plate injury, the adolescent growth spurt, limited thermoregulatory capacity, and maturity-associated variation. Although problems do not ordinarily arise at normal levels of activity, the more frequent and intense training and competition of young athletes today may create conditions under which these risk factors may exert their influence.

Susceptibility to Growth Plate Injury

Growth plate injuries have no counterpart in adult life. Tolerance limits of the growth plate may be exceeded by the mechanical stress of acute injury or by the repetitive physical loading demanded by training regimens in team sports [3]. Physeal injuries can produce permanent injury to the cells in the zone of hypertrophy, resulting in growth disturbance. The resistance of growth plate cartilage to stress is low [4]. It is also more susceptible than articular cartilage to compression and shearing, and than adjacent bone to shear and tension. In addition, the growth plate may be 2–5 times weaker than the surrounding fibrous tissue [5]. Therefore, when disruptive forces are applied to an extremity, failure may occur through the growth plate.

Good epidemiological data on the incidence of physeal injuries in team sports are lacking. However, literature reviews on this topic reveal multiple published case reports and case series that attest to the occurrence of both acute and chronic growth plate injuries in children's team sports [3, 6, 7]. Reports of sport-related physeal injuries resulting in growth disturbance are also reviewed in these papers.

The Adolescent Growth Spurt

The adolescent growth spurt appears to be a time of heightened risk for sports injury. The susceptibility of the growth plate to injury appears to be especially pronounced during periods of rapid growth [8–17]. Research pertaining to the development of physeal cartilage in animals shows a decrease in physeal strength during pubescence [9]. The data on humans are consistent with these findings [10–12]. An increase in the rate of growth at the growth plate is accompanied by structural changes that result in a thicker and more fragile plate [10, 13]. In addition, bone mineralization may lag behind linear growth during the pubescent growth spurt, thus rendering the bone temporarily more porous and subject to injury [14, 15]. Studies of the frequency of physeal and other injuries indicate an increased occurrence of fractures during pubescence [14–17], and a noteworthy association between peak height velocity and peak fracture rate [14].

Results from two injury studies involving gymnasts indicate that high injury risk gymnasts were characterized by advanced competitive levels and rapid growth [18], and the gymnasts between 10 and 14 years of age were significantly more likely to report wrist pain than those who were either above or below this age range [19]. However, both of these latter studies did not compare individual velocities with growth rate.

It is hypothesized that the susceptibility for a variety of musculoskeletal injuries increases during periods of rapid growth because there is an increase in musculoskeletal tightness about the joints, loss of flexibility, and enhanced environment for injury [20]. Longitudinal growth occurs initially in the long bones of the extremities and in the spinal column. The muscle-tendon units that span the bones elongate secondarily in response to bone growth. Thus, during the adolescent growth spurt, these muscle-tendon units may become dramatically tighter thus increasing the risk of both acute and chronic joint-related injury. However, this hypothesis remains controversial [21, 22] and the results of one recent study suggests no loss of flexibility during periods of rapid growth [21].

Limited Thermoregulatory Capacity

Exercising children do not adapt as effectively as adults when exposed to high temperature. This may affect their performance and well-being, and increase the risk for heat-related illness. The thermoregulatory short-comings of children relative to adults during heat and exercise have recently been reviewed [23].

- children gain heat faster from the environment by convection, conduction, and radiation than do adults as a result of their greater surface area-to-body mass ratio than adults;
- children also produce more metabolic heat per mass unit than adults during activities that include walking and running;
- sweating capacity is considerably lower in children than in adults, which reduces their ability to dissipate body heat by evaporation; and
- children acclimatize to exercise in hot weather at a slower rate than adults.

Thus, children will generate more heat for a given activity, yet are less able to dissipate body heat particularly in a hot environment. As children frequently do not feel the urge to drink enough to replenish fluid loss either before or following exercise, they may experience increased risk of dehydration and heat illness [24].

Maturity-Associated Variation

Children of the same chronological age may vary considerably in biological maturity status, and individual differences in maturity status influence measures of growth and performance during childhood and adolescence [23]. For example, there are definite structural, functional, and performance advantages of early-maturity boys in sports requiring size, strength, and power. The fear is that unbalanced competition between early- and late-maturing boys in contact sports such as gridiron football and ice hockey contribute to at least some of the serious injuries in these sports. Although a noninvasive method for estimating maturity status as a basis for grouping young athletes has recently been proposed [25], classification for participation in youth sports continues to rely primarily on chronological age which may add yet another dimension of individual variation. For example, within a single age-group (e.g., 12 years of age), the child who is 12.9 years of age is likely taller, heavier and stronger than the child who is 12.0 years of age, even though both are classified as 12 years of age. Thus, when children are grouped by age, variation is associated with chronological age *per se* and also with differences in biological maturity [23].

Concern for the Health and Safety of Young Athletes

The increased sports involvement of children from an early age and continued through the years of growth, against a background of their apparent vulnerability to injury, gives rise to concern about the risk and severity and long-term effects of injury. Recent data suggest that the risk of pediatric sports injury is high and constitutes a significant public health burden. During 2000–2001, for example, there were an estimated 4.3 million nonfatal sports- and recreation-related injuries treated in US hospital emergency departments [26]. Injury rates for both sexes peaked around adolescence, and were highest for boys. Children 5–14 years of age accounted for nearly 40% of all sports-related injuries [27]. Since only the more serious injuries present to hospital emergency departments, these data reflect only part of the overall injury picture in children's and youth sports. Many more, albeit less severe, injuries are treated in other settings such as healthcare providers' offices and clinics.

Parents need to know about the risks of injuries in children's and youth sports and what they can do to help prevent injury [27]. Indeed, young athletes of all ages and everyone who works with them, whether they be parents, sports medicine personnel, sports governing bodies, or coaches, need to know answers to questions such as the followings: Is the risk of injury greater in some sport activities, or level of activity, than in others? What types of injuries are most common in a given sport? What is the average time lost from injury and what is the risk of permanent impairment? Are some children prone to sports injury? Are some physical, psychological, or sport-related factors associated with an increased risk of injury? Can injury be prevented, and, if so, how? How effective are the preventive measures presently implemented? These are all questions which sports medicine personnel and coaches should be prepared to respond to, and the information should be made readily available to them. Providing this information is an important objective of sports injury epidemiology research.

Epidemiology of Sports Injuries in Children

Sports injury epidemiology studies the distribution and determinants of varying rates of sports injuries for the purpose of identifying and implementing measures to prevent their development and spread [28]. The epidemiologist in sports medicine is concerned with quantifying injury occurrence (how much) with respect to who is affected by injury, where and when injuries occur, and what is their outcome, for the purpose of explaining why and how injuries occur and identifying strategies to control and prevent them. The study of the distribution of varying rates of injuries (i.e. who, where, when, what) is referred to as descriptive epidemiology. The study of the determinants of an exhibited distribution of varying rates of injuries (i.e. why and how) and the effectiveness of selected preventive measures is referred to as analytical epidemiology [28].

The epidemiology of sports injuries in children and youth is an important area of research that has been largely overlooked in the medicine and sport science literature. It deserves serious study, particularly with regards to the identification and analysis of risk factors and preventive measures [29]. However, existing epidemiological research on pediatric sports injuries has already resulted in rule changes, new equipment standards, improved coaching techniques, and better conditioning of athletes [29]. For example, the prohibition of 'spearing' in football, and rules regarding water depth and the racing dive in swimming are examples of how data on deaths and catastrophic injuries can be used to help promote the safety of young athletes. Other preventive measures supported by research include anchoring movable soccer goals to prevent tipping, improved training for high school wrestling coaches, increased awareness of pathogenic weight control in wrestling and gymnastics, use of face shields when batting in baseball, and use of full face shields and rules against pushing or checking from behind in hockey [30].

Purpose and Organization of this Book

The benefits of physical activity for children and youth are substantial. However, growth in sports participation has contributed to an increase in pediatric sports-related injuries. In addition to the immediate healthcare costs, these injuries may have long-term consequences on the musculoskeletal system, resulting in limb dysfunction and a subsequent reduction in levels of physical activity [31]. However, half of all organized sports-related injuries among children can be prevented [32].

The purpose of *Epidemiology of Pediatric Sports Injuries: Team Sports* is to review comprehensively what is known about the distribution and determinants of injury rates in a variety of team sports, and to suggest injury prevention measures and guidelines for further research. This book provides the first comprehensive compilation and critical analysis of epidemiological data over children's team sports: baseball, basketball, gridiron football, ice hockey, rugby, and soccer. The previous volume (*Epidemiology of Pediatric Sports Injuries: Individual Sports*) in Medicine and Sport Science had addressed the epidemiology of injuries in pediatric individual sports.

A common, uniform strategy and evidence-based approach to organizing and interpreting the literature is used in the chapters of both volumes. All the sports-specific chapters are laid out with the same basic headings, so that it is easy for the reader to find common information across chapters. Section headings include, besides the Abstracts and Introductions:
- Incidence of Injury
- Injury Characteristics
- Injury Severity
- Injury Risk Factors
- Suggestions for Injury Prevention
- Suggestions for Further Research

In each sport-specific chapter, an epidemiological picture has been systematically developed from the data available in prospective cohort, retrospective cohort, case-control, and cross-sectional studies (i.e. denominator-based designs). From this picture, it became possible to suggest preventive measures which seemed at least reasonable, given the level of evidence available, and to suggest needed areas for further research. A chapter titled 'Injury Prevention and Future Research' that addresses individual and team sports is included at the end of both volumes to provide a more global, across-sport examination of the literature identifying risk factors and prevention strategies for injury in child and adolescent sports.

Sport scientists and healthcare professionals will find *Epidemiology of Pediatric Sports Injuries* – both *Vol. 48: Individual Sports* and *Vol. 49: Team Sports* – useful in identifying problem areas in which appropriate preventive measures can be initiated to reduce the risk and severity of injuries. They will also want to use these volumes as a resource for research initiatives in the epidemiology of children's sports injuries. Sports administrators and coaches will find these books a thought-provoking reference that spurs discussion and encourages changes in the rules, equipment standards, coaching techniques, and athlete conditioning programs they use. Finally, these volumes will provide these individuals with current information on the epidemiology of pediatric sports injuries so that they, in turn, can inform parents about the risks of injury in children's sports and how they can help their children avoid or limit these risks.

References

1   Maffulli N: Children in sport: Questions and controversies; in Maffulli N (ed): Color Atlas and Text of Sports Medicine in Childhood and Adolescence. London, Mosby-Wolfe, 1995, pp 7–14.
2   Pensgaard AM, Roberts GC: The relationship between motivational climate, perceived ability and sources of distress among elite athletes. J Sports Sci 2000;18:191–200.
3   Caine DJ: Growth plate injury and bone growth: An update. Ped Exerc Sci 1990;2:209–229.
4   Micheli LJ: Pediatric and adolescent sports injury: Recent trends; in Pandolf KP (ed): Exercise and Sport Science Reviews. New York, Macmillan, 1986, pp 359–374.
5   Larson RL, McMahon RO: The epiphyses and the childhood athlete. JAMA 1966;196:607–612.
6   Caine DJ, Lindner K: Growth plate injury: A threat to young distance runners? Phys Sportsmed 1984;12:118–124.
7   Caine D: Injury and growth; in Sands WA, Caine DJ, Borms J (eds): Scientific Aspects of Women's Gymnastics. Med Sport Sci. Basel, Karger, 2003, vol 45, pp 46–71.
8   Ogden JA: Skeletal Injury in the Child. New York, Springer, 2000.
9   Bright RW, Burstein AH, Elmore SM: Epiphyseal-plate cartilage: A biomechanical and histological analysis of failure modes. J Bone Jt Surg (Am) 1974;56:688–703.
10 Alexander CJ: Effect of growth rate on the strength of the growth plate-shaft function. Skeletal Radiol 1976;1:67–76.
11 Morsher E: Strength and morphology of growth cartilage under hormonal influence of puberty. Reconstr Surg Traumatol 1968;10:1–96.
12 Speer DP, Braun JK: The biomechanical basis of growth plate injuries. Phys Sportsmed 1985; 13:72–78.

13 Aldridge MJ: Overuse injuries of the distal radial growth epiphysis; in Hoshizaki BT, Salmela JH, Petiot B (eds): Diagnostics, Treatment and Analysis of Gymnastic Talent. Montreal, Sports Psyche Editions, 1987, pp 25–30.

14 Bailey DA, Wedge JH, McCulloch RG, Martin AD, Bernardson SC: Epidemiology of fractures of the distal end of the radius in children as associated with growth. J Bone Jt Surg [Am] 1989;71: 1225–1231.

15 Bradford DS: Vertebral osteochondrosis (Scheuermann's kyphosis). Clin Orthop 1981;158:83–90.

16 Peterson CA, Peterson HA: Analysis of the incidence of injuries to the epiphyseal growth plate. J Trauma 1972;12:275–281.

17 Benton JW: Epiphyseal fracture in sports. Phys Sportsmed 1982;10:63–71.

18 Caine D, Cochrane B, Caine C, Zemper E: An epidemiological investigation of injuries affecting young competitive female gymnasts. Am J Sports Med 1989;17:811–820.

19 DiFiori JP, Puffer JC, Aish B, Dorey F: Wrist pain in young gymnasts: Frequency and effects on training over 1 year. Clin J Sport Med 2002;12:348–353.

20 Micheli LJ: Overuse injuries in children's sports. The growth factor. Orthop Clin North Am 1983;14:337–360.

21 Feldman D, Shrier I, Rossignol M, Abenhaim L: Adolescent growth is not associated with changes in flexibility. Clin J Sport Med 1999;9:24–29.

22 Micheli LJ: Is adolescent growth associated with changes in flexibility. Clin J Sport Med 2000;10:76.

23 Malina RM, Bouchard C, Bar-Or O: Growth, Maturation, and Physical Activity (ed2), Human Kinetics, 2004, pp 267–273.

24 Walker SM, Casa DJ, Levrealt ML, Psathas E, Sparrow SL, Decher DR: Children participating in summer sports camps are chronically dehydrated. Med Sci Sports Exerc 2004;36(suppl 5): S180–S181.

25 Mirwald RL, Baxter-Jones ADG, Bailey DA, Beunen GP: An assessment of maturity from anthropometric measurements. Med Sci Sports Exerc 2002;34:689–694.

26 Centers for Disease Control and Prevention Morbidity and Mortality Weekly Report: Non-fatal sports- and recreation-related injuries treated in emergency departments, United States, July 2000–June 2001. MMWR Weekly 2002;51(33):736–740. Available from URL: http://www.cdc.gov/mmwr/preview/mmwrhtml/mm5133a2.htm [Accessed on July 31, 2004].

27 National Safe Kids Campaign: Get into the game: A national survey of parents' knowledge, attitudes and self-reported behaviors concerning sports safety. Press Release, May 4, 2000. Available from URL: http://www.safekids.org/[Accessed on July 31, 2004].

28 Caine C, Caine D, Lindner K: The epidemiologic approach; in Caine D, Caine C, Lindner K (eds): Epidemiology of Sports Injuries. Champaign, Human Kinetics, 1996, pp 1–13.

29 Mueller F, Blyth C: Epidemiology of injuries in children. Clin Sports Med 1982;1:343–352.

30 Cantu RC, Mueller FO: Fatalities and catastrophic injuries in high school and college sports, 1982–97. Phys Sportsmed 1999;27:35.

31 Arendt EA: Specific injury locations – Overview; in Garrett WE, Lester GE, McGown J, Kirkendall DT (eds): Women's Health in Sports and Exercise. Rosemont, American Academy of Orthopedic Surgeons, 2001, pp 85–86.

32 National Safe Kids Campaign: Injury Facts. Available from URL: http://www.safekids.org/[Accessed on July 31, 2004].

Nicola Maffulli, MD, MS, PhD, FRCS (Orth)
Department of Trauma and Orthopedic Surgery
Keele University School of Medicine
Stoke on Trent ST4 7QB (UK)
Tel. +44 1782 554 999, Fax +44 1782 412 236, E-Mail n.maffulli@keele.ac.uk

Maffulli N, Caine DJ (eds): Epidemiology of Pediatric Sports Injuries: Team Sports.
Med Sport Sci. Basel, Karger, 2005, vol 49, pp 9–30

··························

Baseball Injuries

Stephen Lyman, Glenn S. Fleisig

American Sports Medicine Institute, Birmingham, Ala., USA

Abstract

Objective: To identify the frequency of injury in youth baseball, risk factors for these injuries, and possible prevention measures to reduce the frequency or severity of these injuries. **Data Sources:** Information was collected from all known epidemiologic and intervention studies published in the peer-reviewed medical and scientific literature as it applies to youth baseball injuries. **Main Results:** The frequency and severity of youth baseball injuries have remained relatively consistent over time. Risk factors for many injuries have been understudied and the study designs used for much of this research have been less than optimal. Several effective prevention measures have been identified, such as batting helmets, face shields, softer baseballs, and breakaway bases. **Conclusions:** Baseball is a relatively safe sport compared to many contact sports, but injuries do still occur. Future research should focus on determining the optimum pitching motion for both arm safety and performance, as well as systematically studying other potential safety improvements such as restrictions against breaking pitches.

Introduction

In the United States, over 20 million people play organized baseball per year, a vast majority of whom are children and teenagers [1]. Although baseball is believed to be one of the safest team sports in which athletes participate [2, 3], the sheer number of players makes any relatively frequent injuries important to prevent.

The purpose of this chapter is to review the history of published peer-reviewed literature on juvenile baseball injuries. The literature review consists of all published English language articles evaluating the epidemiology of baseball injuries in children since 1966 as identified through Medline (descriptors: baseball OR pitching AND child OR adolescent OR youth). The ancestry approach was used to identify additional relevant articles not arising from the database search. Only those articles that focused on the frequency and determinants of baseball injury were included in this review.

Many previously published studies of baseball injuries in children suffer from the methodological problems described by Walter and Hart [4]. These studies used varying definitions of injury, making cross-study comparison difficult. In many studies, injury rates were not calculated based on exposure, but rather on participation, even though exposure may differ for each participant. Nearly all reports of youth baseball injury were retrospective, case, or case series. Few studies have used cross-sectional or prospective designs. Only population-based retrospective or prospective cohort studies will be evaluated in this chapter. The volume of case studies and case series is enormous, but of little use in the understanding of the frequency and determinants of baseball injury in children.

Incidence of Injury

Injury Rates

A comparison of injury rates in youth [3, 5, 6, 10, 12, 16, 17] and high school [7–9, 11, 13–15] are shown in table 1. Overall, the rates of injury in youth and high school baseball are lower than other sports played by children and adolescents, but they still represent a significant cause of injury and potential long-term disability among the participants [18], particularly among pitchers [19–28].

Youth Baseball

For this review, youth baseball was defined as pre-high school recreational league play such as 'Little League'. The original study of the epidemiology of baseball injuries in children by Hale [10] in 1960 retrospectively reviewed insurance claims over a 5-year period; finding 2.0 injuries per 100 participants. This is likely an underestimate since only athletes making an insurance claim were included as injuries. Many more athletes were likely injured without seeking medical care through the insurance system.

More than 40 years later, Marshall, et al. [12] replicated and expanded upon Dr. Hale's original research by looking at the compensated insurance claims in Little League Baseball. This study demonstrated a very low rate of compensated insurance claims with only 0.62 injuries per 1,000 player-seasons, a substantial reduction from Dr. Hale's original estimates. Either youth baseball has become much safer or league insurance claims are much less common due to private insurance coverage for players.

Table 1. Comparison of injury rates in baseball

Study (year)	Duration in years	Design	Data source	Participants	Injuries	Rate per 100 athletes (unless otherwise noted)
Youth						
Hale (1960) [10]	5	Retrospective	Insurance records	771,810	15,444	2.0
Chambers (1979) [5]	1	Prospective	Survey	740	2	0.27
Zaricznyj et al. (1980) [17]	1	Retrospective	Survey	137	13	9.5
Pasternack et al. (1996) [3]	1	Prospective	Survey	2,861	81	2.8
Cheng et al. (2000) [6]	2	Prospective	ER records	64,075[a]	76	0.74[b]
Radelet et al. (2002) [16]	2	Prospective	Survey	534	117	0.17[c]
Marshall et al. (2003) [12]	3	Retrospective	Insurance records	6,744,240[d]	4,233	0.62[e]
High School						
Garrick and Requa (1978) [8]	2	Prospective	Survey	249	46	0.18[c]
Grana (1979) [9]	1	Retrospective	Survey	1,969	29	1.47
Lowe et al. (1987) [11]	1	Retrospective	Survey	256	3	1.22
Martin et al. (1987) [13]	1[f]	Prospective	Survey	148	8	5.4
McLain and Reynolds (1989) [14]	1	Prospective	Survey	68	10	15.0
DuRant et al. (1992) [7]	1	Prospective	Survey	108	21	19.4
Powell and Barber-Foss (2000) [15]	3	Prospective	Surveillance system	2,167	861	13.2

[a]Catchment population ages 10–19 for emergency room visits.
[b]per 1,000 adolescents ages 10–19.
[c]per 1,000 athlete-exposures (A-E).
[d]Count of number of seasons during the three year follow-up period.
[e]per 1,000 athlete-seasons.
[f]Followed one high school baseball tournament.

Several smaller studies demonstrated widely disparate injury rates in youth baseball from 0.27 per 100 athletes to 9.5 per 100 athletes [3, 5, 6, 16, 17]. In 2000, Cheng et al. [6] reported 76 baseball-related emergency room visits among adolescents over 2 years in Washington, DC. This translated to an injury rate of 0.74 per 1,000 adolescents, but not all DC area youths played baseball, so this rate is not directly comparable to other rates presented here.

Radelet et al. [16] found an injury rate of 0.17 per 1,000 athletic exposures (A-E). Since this study used A-E rather than a person-based rate denominator, the results are not directly comparable to other studies among children in these ages. Nonetheless, it is likely the most representative study of the true injury rates in youth baseball.

High School Baseball

Garrick and Requa [8] published the first study of high school baseball injuries in 1978. This was the earliest baseball epidemiology study that used A-E as a rate denominator rather than a count of athletes. The rate of 0.18 per 1,000 A-E translates to a rate of 9.2 injuries per 100 athletes per year (table 1). This is very similar to the rate found by Radalet et al. [16] for youth baseball using very similar methodology. Subsequently, two retrospective studies found injury rates of 1.2–1.5 per 100 athletes [9, 11] and several prospective studies found injury rates from 5.4 (in a single tournament) to 19.4 per 100 athletes [7, 13–15]. A study by Powell and Barber-Foss [15] followed 2,167 high school players prospectively for 3 seasons, making it the largest study of the incidence of high school baseball injury to date. The finding of an injury rate of 13.2 per 100 athletes is in line with previous prospective studies, but may represent the most stable estimate available for the true incidence of baseball injuries in high school athletes due to the large sample size.

The retrospective follow-up studies of high school players have found injury rates of less than 2 per 100 athletes while the prospective follow-up studies of these players have found injury rates of 9 or greater per 100 athletes. This gross disparity suggests that a uniform definition of injury must be identified and that retrospective studies are likely substantially limited by recall bias and under-ascertainment.

Pitching Injuries

Approximately 25% of youth baseball players participate as pitchers. Pitching is the primary defensive tool in the sport of baseball, and it requires the repetition of a dynamic arm motion during which the pitcher delivers the ball to the batter. Several studies have found high rates of mild to moderate elbow and shoulder pain in youth and adolescent pitchers. These injuries are believed to be a result of overuse of the affected joints. Furthermore, continued overuse is believed to eventually result in serious injury or arm-related disability in some pitchers [18].

Table 2 summarizes the findings of studies of elbow and shoulder injury in pitchers published between 1965 and 2002 [19–28]. In 1965, Adams conducted the seminal epidemiologic study on this issue [19]. This study identified injuries as pitcher self-report of elbow soreness while pitching. Adams compared 3 groups of male children: pitchers, baseball players who did not pitch, and healthy boys who did not play baseball. The frequency of arm pain was highest in pitchers. Subsequent studies of American youth and high school players have demonstrated a prevalence of elbow pain between 18 and 29% [22, 24, 27, 28] and an incidence of elbow pain of 26% among youth players and 58% among high school players [20, 21, 23, 25, 26]. Shoulder pain has not been studied as frequently with a prevalence of 29% in single study of 9–18-year-old boys [28] and an incidence of 32–35% in two recent studies by Lyman et al. [25, 26].

A Taiwan Little League study evaluated all pitchers participating in the 1980 Taiwan Little League championship tournament [23]. Injury was defined as a complaint of elbow soreness during the tournament. This study evaluated a specific location of elbow injury and found that 41% of the pitchers experienced tenderness over the medial epicondylar region of the elbow during the tournament. Another Asian study among Japanese High School pitchers was conducted during the Japanese High School Baseball Association national championship [27]. Injury was defined as a self-reported history of shoulder or elbow pain, and a frequency of 38% was found for each.

All of the above studies used radiographic comparison of pitchers' throwing elbows to their non-throwing elbows. The initial study in 1965 identified radiographic changes in the arms of 95% of the pitchers compared with 11% in the group of non-pitching baseball players [19]. Subsequent studies have found radiographic changes in 4–95% of the elbows of youth and high school pitchers [6, 20–22, 24, 27, 28]. In no study was the radiographic identification of elbow abnormality correlated with elbow pain. Individual interpretation of the radiographs may explain part of the differences identified. The studies also used inconsistent definitions of *abnormal* when reviewing radiographs. No study examined the shoulders of these pitchers with radiographs.

Two recent studies found incidence rates of self-reported elbow pain in more than 25% of pitchers and self-reported shoulder pain in more than 30% of pitchers [25, 26]. These studies used a prospective design with pitcher interviews occurring after each game pitched, improving on previous designs in which pitchers were interviewed only after the tournament or season was completed. This reduces recall bias in this young population. Radiographic exams were not

Table 2. Studies of elbow and shoulder injury in pitchers

Study (year)	Level, Location	Design	N	Age in years	Affected joint	Frequency measure	Per cent reporting pain	Per cent with X-ray changes[a]
Youth Leagues								
Adams, (1965) [19]	Various, Calif., USA	Retrospective	80	9–14	Elbow	Prevalence	45	95
Gugenheim et al. (1976) [22]	Little League, Tex., USA	Retrospective	595	11–12	Elbow	Prevalence	18	28
Larson et al. (1976) [24]	Little League, Oreg., USA	Retrospective	120	11–12	Elbow	Prevalence	18	95
Albright et al. (1978) [20]	Little League, Conn., USA	Prospective	54	11–12	Both	Incidence	44	n.a.
Hang (1979) [23]	Little League, Taiwan	Prospective	112	11–12	Elbow	Incidence	69	62
Lyman et al. (2001) [25]	Various, Ala., USA	Prospective	298	9–12	Elbow Shoulder	Incidence	26 32	n.a.
Lyman et al. (2002) [26]	Various, Ala., USA	Prospective	488	9–14	Elbow Shoulder	Incidence	28 35	n.a.
Mixed								
Torg et al. (1972) [28]	Boys' Club, Pa., USA	Retrospective	49	9–18	Elbow Shoulder	Prevalence	29 29	4 n.a.
High School								
Grana and Rashkin (1980) [21]	High School, USA	Prospective	73	15–18	Elbow	Incidence	58	56
Ochi et al. (1994) [27]	High School, Japan	Retrospective	130	15–18	Elbow Shoulder	Prevalence	38 38	43 n.a.

[a]Regardless of pain status.

conducted in this study because previous research had shown no consistent relationship between radiographic abnormalities and arm pain.

Injury Characteristics

Injury Onset

Injuries to fielders and batters tend to be acute traumatic injuries due to contact with the ball, bat, another player, the ground, or a base [29]. On the other hand, injuries to pitchers tend to be the result of cumulative microtrauma through the repetitive throwing motion [30, 31].

Injury Location

Head, Face, and Torso

Injuries to the head, face, and torso are relatively uncommon in baseball compared to contact sports such as football, ice hockey, or lacrosse, but they represent an often severe result of baseball participation with fractures, concussion, traumatic brain injury, and sudden death all possible. Marshall et al. [12] reported a risk of facial injury in youth players at 4.1 per 100,000 player-seasons based on insurance claims data with Little League Baseball. A discussion of traumatic brain injury and *commotio cordis* appears in the Catastrophic Injury section of this chapter.

Upper Extremity

Injuries to the upper extremity are very common in baseball pitchers and other players as well. The incidence of elbow and shoulder injury in youth baseball has been estimated at 26–35 per 100 pitchers per season [25, 26]. The definition of injury in these studies has usually been 'pain' in the elbow or shoulder during or after pitching. While this does not necessarily reflect a medical problem, it does cause discomfort to children participating in a voluntary activity. Perhaps, more importantly, joint pain may be an early indicator of a developing serious overuse injury.

Clinically meaningful elbow and shoulder problems in pitchers have been euphemistically described as 'Little League Elbow' and 'Little League Shoulder' [23, 32]. This is an unfortunate implication of Little League Baseball, Inc., which has done more research in an effort to prevent arm injuries in youth pitchers than any other youth baseball organization, funding many of the studies presented in this chapter. For the purposes of this discussion, Little League Elbow will be referred to as medial epicondylitis and Little League Shoulder will be referred to as a widening of the proximal humeral epiphysis, both of which are the more medically correct terms.

Lower Extremity

Lower extremity injuries are relatively uncommon among youth baseball players [31], but become more common as age increases and the level of play becomes more aggressive [15]. Ankle and knee injuries are frequent as a result of sliding at higher age levels [33].

Action or Activity

Pitching Injuries

Pitching is likely the most injury-prone activity at all levels of baseball due to the cumulative microtrauma to the elbow and shoulder, but it is possibly most risky among youth players because of their immature skeletons. The severe pitching injuries seen in high school, college, and professional pitchers are likely due to cumulative trauma that began as children.

Batting Injuries

Danis et al. [34] conducted a study examining the rate of batting injuries, but restricted this to only facial injuries. This study compared youth players using a face shield while batting versus players not wearing a face shield while batting. The results of this comparison will be discussed further in 'practical applications'. However, for the purposes of reporting a background incidence, 5.3 per 100 athletes reported a facial injury while batting during a single youth season. The nature and severity of the injuries was not disclosed.

Base-Running Injuries

Most injuries which occur during base-running are the result of sliding into bases. Previous research into sliding injuries has focused on comparisons of breakaway bases versus traditional bases and has included youth and adult players as well as baseball and softball leagues. Therefore, the rates of sliding injury found in these studies are not directly applicable to youth baseball, because baseball and softball as well as adults and children have different rates of injuries. These studies will be discussed in 'practical applications'.

Fielding Injuries

No previous studies of fielding injuries are available for review. Fielding injuries are thought to usually occur due to contact with the ball, the ground, another fielder, or a fence [29].

Chronometry

Radalet et al. [16] found a significant difference in the risk of injury between games and practice with injuries in games four times more common than injuries during practice. Powell and Barber-Foss [35] found a similar relationship for the risk of traumatic brain injury in high school players between games and practices.

Injury Severity

Most baseball injuries among children and adolescents are not severe. Abrasions are the most common injury types followed by fractures, sprains/ strains, and lacerations. With the exception of sprains of the ligaments or tendons, all of these injuries should heal completely with little or no residual deficit. However, if left untreated, a ligament or tendon injury may cause continued pain with participation or may contribute to a loss of playing ability.

Injury Type

Previous studies of the types of injuries in youth baseball have found that abrasions are the most common type of injury [10, 36], while fractures, sprains/strains, and lacerations follow. A single report of high school injury types reported fractures, sprains, and lacerations as having nearly equal frequency [11]. The utility of this information is suspect, because studies often used differing definitions of 'injury'. Some studies required only self-report of injury [13, 22, 24–26], some required a hospital visit [6], while some required an insurance claim [10, 12]. Since abrasions might not require medical attention from a trained health professional or an insurance claim, these are likely greatly under-reported in some studies. Also, since these injuries are common, but mild, they may not be an important part of the safety of youth baseball.

Medical epicondylitis, or pain and inflammation in the medial aspect of the elbow joint, is a common injury among youth pitchers likely because of the secondary ossification centers present in the young elbow. Between the ages of 2 and 11, no less than 6 of these secondary bone growth centers develop in the elbow joint, fusing to the ends of the long bones between the ages of 13 and 17 [37]. These unattached bony growths make the young elbow particularly vulnerable to injury because the elbow does not have the stability of a skeletally mature athlete's elbow.

Widening of the proximal humeral epiphysis occurs from repetitive pitching in the skeletally immature athlete [37–39]. This widening of the growth plate in the proximal end of the humeral shaft may result in pain during or after pitching and may result in deformity if left untreated [32]. A less common, but more traumatic upper extremity injury is the fracture of the humeral shaft due to rotational forces during throwing [40].

Catastrophic Injury

Commotio cordis is the most common cause of injury death as a result of playing baseball [41–43]. Spinal and severe head injuries are much less common in baseball than in contact sports such as football or ice hockey [35].

Maron et al. [43] reported on 128 cases of *commotio cordis*, which is cardiac arrest as a result of blunt trauma to the chest, from all causes in the USA over a more than 20-year period. Of these cases, 107 died as a result of their injury with 53 of the cases the result of a blow from a thrown or batted baseball. The median age of these victims was 14 years.

Powell and Barber-Foss [35] conducted a study of traumatic brain injury in high school athletes, finding that baseball had the lowest risk of traumatic brain injury among the major sports (baseball, basketball, football, soccer, and wrestling) with a rate of 0.05 per 1,000 A-E. Nine of the fifteen traumatic brain injuries reported among baseball players occurred during a collision with another player, 3 with a bat, 2 with a pitch, and 1 from sliding. Fewer than half of the athletes missed more than a week of participation and none missed more than 3 weeks.

Time Loss

Time loss from practice or competition has been evaluated in only two studies, both among high school athletes. Garrick and Requa [8] found that 27% of baseball players lost at least 5 days of practice or games to injury. Powell and Barber-Foss [35] found that the median time lost due to traumatic brain injury for baseball players was 3 days with no player requiring more than 3 weeks to recover.

Clinical Outcome

Francis et al. [18] reported that 15% of a sample of 398 male college students who pitched in youth baseball felt their ability to throw in college was hindered or hampered by pain, tenderness, or limitation of movement as a result of their youth baseball pitching. Also, 58% reported having experienced arm pain at some point during their youth league years. Radiographic evaluation found no differences between those who reported pain and those who did not. This is not surprising since none of the studies that evaluated radiographic changes have linked these changes to injury. Nevertheless, this study suggests a potential for sports-related disability that is associated with youth baseball pitching and continues into adulthood. No similar study of the long-term effects of baseball participation has been conducted for other baseball injuries.

Injury Risk Factors

Compared to research in other medical research areas, the risk factor literature on youth baseball injuries is relatively sparse. However, some clear patterns have emerged. Table 3 presents the intrinsic and extrinsic risk factors identified, or at least explored, in the youth baseball injury literature [3, 5, 7, 10, 12–16, 20, 21, 25, 26, 29, 36, 42–47]. Levels of evidence were subjectively graded on a four-point scale – high (multiple studies confirming a strong association), moderate (at least one study confirming a modest association), fair (at least one study confirming a modest association, but with at least one other study with a null finding), and low (small association found in only one study, but contradicted in other studies).

Intrinsic Factors

Intrinsic risk factors are usually not modifiable (e.g. age, race, sex), which makes them of limited utility when attempting to intervene to prevent injury. However, those that are significantly associated with the risk of injury should be accounted for in analyses of modifiable risk factors. Fortunately, in baseball there are several modifiable intrinsic risk factors, particularly with regard to the motions players use to complete tasks such as batting, throwing, sliding, fielding, and pitching.

Non-Pitchers

Many intrinsic injury risk factors for non-pitchers are similar to those in pitchers, but have not been explored as thoroughly. High school injury rates are consistently higher than youth baseball injury rates. This suggests that level of play increases the risk of injury as bigger, stronger, and more aggressive players play the game with faster throws, harder hits, and faster running. High school players have a greater risk of injuring their lower extremities than younger players, which may be attributed to a more aggressive style of play [15, 31] (table 3). However, younger players are more likely to suffer injuries from pitched or batted balls [10, 29, 36].

Pitchers

Age, Height, and Weight. Lyman et al. [25] found that among 9–12-year-old pitchers, the risk of elbow pain increased with age and body weight [25]. The association with age is likely due to the development of additional secondary ossification centers about the elbow between the ages of 9 and 12 years. Conversely, height was associated with a decreased risk of elbow pain, which may be an indication of skeletal maturity with those secondary ossification centers having fused. With regard to the shoulder, age was associated with a

Table 3. Risk factors for baseball injuries in youth players

Risk factor	Description of association	Level of evidence
Intrinsic risk factors:		
Field players:		
Older players [3, 5, 7, 13–16]	High school players have higher injury rates than youth players across prospective studies, but this has not been demonstrated within a single population.	Fair
Younger players [10, 29, 36]	Younger players have consistently been demonstrated to be at increased risk of injury from pitched or batted balls.	High
Pitchers:		
Age [25, 26]	Increasing age was associated with an increased risk of elbow pain in a single prospective study of youth pitchers. A subsequent evaluation of youth pitchers did not demonstrate a clear relationship.	Moderate
Body weight [25]	Increasing weight was associated with increased risk of elbow pain in a single prospective study of youth pitchers.	Moderate
Height [25]	Increasing height was associated with a decreased risk of elbow pain and an increased risk of shoulder pain in a single prospective study of youth pitchers.	Moderate
Pitching motion [20, 21, 26]	Sidearm pitching motion was associated with an increased risk of elbow pain in a single small prospective study of youth pitchers. No other studies have demonstrated a relationship.	Fair
Self-satisfaction with performance [25]	Pitchers less satisfied with their pitching performance were more likely to report elbow and shoulder pain in a single prospective study of youth pitchers.	Moderate
Extrinsic risk factors:		
Field players:		
Baseball hardness [12, 42, 43–45]	Both animal and clinical studies have demonstrated that harder baseballs result in more injuries and a higher risk of *commotio cordis.*	High
Fixed bases [46, 47]	Intervention trials have demonstrated that fixed bases result in far more lower extremity injuries than breakaway bases.	High

Table 3 (continued)

Risk factor	Description of association	Level of evidence
Pitchers (youth only):		
Pitches thrown per game [25, 26]	Two prospective cohort studies have demonstrated an increased risk of shoulder pain with increasing game pitch counts.	High
Pitches thrown per season [25, 26]	Two prospective cohort studies have demonstrated an increased risk of elbow and shoulder pain with increasing season pitch counts.	High
Curveball use [25, 26]	A single prospective cohort study demonstrated a 50% increased risk of shoulder pain with curveball use, but another study showed no association.	Fair
Slider use [25, 26]	A single prospective cohort study demonstrated an 80% increased risk of elbow pain with slider use, but another study showed no association.	Fair
Change-up use [25, 26]	Two prospective studies have demonstrated a consistent, but nonsignificant 30% decreased risk of shoulder pain with change up use.	Moderate
Weightlifting [25]	A single prospective cohort study found an association between weightlifting and elbow pain in youth pitchers.	Moderate
Playing baseball outside of organized league play [25]	A single prospective cohort study found an association between playing outside of organized league play and increased risk of elbow pain.	Moderate

nonsignificant decreased risk of shoulder pain, while height was associated with a nonsignificant increased risk of shoulder pain.

Pitching Motion. Albright et al. [20] found that youth pitchers who threw with a sidearm motion rather than overhand motion were at increased risk of elbow pain. Other aspects of the pitching motion were evaluated, but none were found to be significant.

Grana and Rashkin [21] attempted to qualify the pitching motion in high school pitchers using three separate indices: orientation of the hand to the shoulder, velocity, and pitching style. None of these indices were associated with current elbow pain except among those pitchers with previous injury, who were more likely to have a loose orientation and moderate velocity. The investigators concluded that this association was likely a result of compensation for the previous injury rather than a cause of the current injury. While this study predates modern biomechanical analysis of the pitching motion, it provided the first look at the motion as a risk factor for arm injury in young players.

Lyman et al. [26] attempted to use a qualitative measure of the pitching motion developed by the American Sports Medicine Institute (ASMI) to correlate the pitching motion with elbow or shoulder problems. The only correlation found that mechanical 'flaws' decreased the risk of elbow and shoulder pain. This correlation may be due to limitations in the study, including qualitative analysis of pitching mechanics from video, the skill level of the subjects, limitations to the normative ASMI model, and the sample size.

Research conducted at ASMI has quantified shoulder and elbow kinetics (i.e. forces and torques) with implications for injury mechanisms [48, 49]. Proper pitching kinematics (i.e. motions) have also been quantified [50, 51], and a relationship between improper kinematics and increased kinetics has been demonstrated [52]. A recent study found that there are few differences between youth and adult pitching kinematics, implying that a youth pitcher may be able to learn proper mechanics at a young age [53].

Self-Satisfaction. The role of psychology in the self-report of injury should not be overlooked when conducting research in pediatric athletes. Lyman et al. [25] asked pitchers to rate their performance in each game pitched. Their level of self-satisfaction was inversely related to their likelihood of claiming to have experienced arm pain as a result of pitching in that game. Whether this represented using pain as an excuse for performance or reason for performance is unknown. There was no association between perceived performance and actual performance (e.g. runs allowed or being the winning pitcher).

Extrinsic Factors
Non-Pitchers
The extrinsic risk factors associated with injuries in non-pitchers are primarily related to the environment in which the game is played: the hardness of the baseball, the rigidity of bases, and the protective equipment used while batting, fielding, and base-running.

Baseball Hardness. Impact trauma from the baseball or a baseball bat is a common cause of injury during competition. Efforts have been made to decrease the hardness of baseballs used among younger players in an effort to reduce the frequency of contusions, fractures, and most importantly, *commotio cordis* [12, 44]. Despite the laboratory-based efficacy of these softer baseballs at reducing the likelihood of impact trauma, 2 cases of *commotio cordis* have been reported after chest wall contact with a reduced-impact baseball [43]. Also, these reduced impact baseballs may increase the severity of eye injury based on laboratory testing of the deformity characteristics of these balls [45].

Fixed Bases. Sliding injuries due to contact with the fixed base are relatively common and can be quite serious with ankle fractures and sprains and knee sprains being common injuries during sliding or base-running [46, 47]. Efforts to teach proper sliding technique may have limited utility [34, 47], but as has been demonstrated time and again in all areas of disease and injury prevention, it is more effective to change the environment than change human behavior. Breakaway bases provide just such an environmental change and have been proven effective [46, 47].

Pitchers

Extrinsic risk factors for injuries to pitchers apart from those associated with reducing the risk of injury from batted balls have focused primarily on the types of pitches thrown and the number of pitches thrown.

Pitch Counts. Gugenheim et al. [22] calculated the average pitches per inning for approximately 25% of the pitchers in the study. No association was found between average pitches per inning and self-reported elbow pain. The authors stated that this was probably because those pitchers who threw more pitches per inning were not used as often as those with better control.

The first study conducted by Lyman et al. [25] looked at the number of pitches thrown in a game and during the season among pitchers aged 9–12 [25]. There was no significant association between pitches thrown during a game and elbow pain. However, a highly significant dose-response relationship was found for shoulder pain as game pitches increased. The second study conducted by Lyman et al. [26] replicated the methods of the first study with a larger sample size, with a broader age range (9–14), and from a larger geographic area and found a similar association with regard to game pitches [26].

The total number of pitches thrown in a season told a different story. Pitchers who threw a high number of pitches over the course of the season in the first Lyman study had a significantly increased risk of elbow pain and a significantly decreased risk of shoulder pain [25]. The decreased risk of shoulder pain was thought to be due to survivorship, in which pitchers who had low cumulative pitch counts were those who stopped pitching or reduced their workload to avoid shoulder pain. Replication of this study did not yield the same results with the risk of both elbow and shoulder pain increasing as cumulative season pitches increased [26].

Pitch Types. Grana and Rashkin's [21] study of high school pitchers stated that approximately 80% of the pitches thrown were breaking pitches (i.e. pitches that are thrown with the intention of deceiving the hitter through downward or horizontal movement of the ball during flight). No attempt was made to examine the relationship between these pitches and risk of elbow pain. Lyman et al. [25] considered pitch types in both studies. In the first study, the sinkerball or forkball was found to be associated with a nonsignificant (p = 0.06) elevated risk of elbow pain. In a stratified analysis, older pitchers who threw a change-up had a significantly decreased risk of elbow pain. In the second study by Lyman et al. [26] change-up use showed a general decrease in the risk of shoulder pain, but it was not a significant association. However, use of the curveball was associated with a significant increased risk of shoulder pain and use of the slider was associated with a significant increased risk of elbow pain.

Research has been conducted to compare the biomechanics of the fastball and the two most common breaking pitches, the curveball and the slider. The results indicate that the curveball may be the most difficult and dangerous pitch to learn, as it requires large forces and torques at the elbow and shoulder like a fastball and slider, but with significantly different mechanics [54, 55].

Other factors. Two other risk factors for elbow pain identified by Lyman et al. [25] are weightlifting and playing baseball outside of the league. The weightlifting association is of little utility, because it is unknown what type of weightlifting was performed and how frequently. There may be arm-strengthening exercises that are not detrimental to elbow health in pitchers. Playing baseball outside of the league likely elevated the pitch counts beyond those recorded in the study, contributing to further overuse of the elbow. This finding could be extended to pitching in multiple leagues, which may double the pitch counts for pitchers.

Suggestions for Injury Prevention

Several studies have demonstrated injury prevention tools for youth baseball players through either equipment changes or behavioral modifications. Table 4 presents the injury prevention methods previously studied that may improve youth baseball safety [12, 26, 29, 35, 44–47, 56]. Levels of evidence were subjectively graded on a four-point scale – high (multiple studies confirming a strong protective effect), moderate (at least one study confirming a modest protective effect), fair (at least one study confirming a modest protective effect, but with at least one other study with a null finding), and low (small protective effect found in one study, but contradicted in other studies).

Batting Helmets and Face Guards
Batting helmets have been in use in youth and high school baseball for decades. Seminal work done by Dr. Creighton Hale of Little League Baseball, Inc.

Table 4. Interventions for increasing youth baseball safety

Intervention	Safety advantage	Level of evidence
Batting helmets [29, 56]	Batting helmets offer significant protection from head injury and are used at all levels of organized baseball.	High
Face guards [12, 35]	Face guards lower the risk of facial and dental injury and have become increasingly accepted at lower levels of youth baseball.	High
Safety baseballs [12, 44, 45]	Safety baseballs are softer than traditional baseballs. They reduce the risk of contusions and other injuries associated with baseballs, but the current designs may increase the risk of eye injury due to their deformity characteristics.	Moderate
Breakaway bases [46, 47]	Several intervention trials have demonstrated a greatly reduced risk of lower extremity injury from sliding.	High
Sliding techniques [24]	Reducing sliding injuries through education has been largely ineffective – breakaway bases represent a much more effective intervention.	Low
Pitching limits [25, 26]	Pitch limits have not been instituted at any level of youth competition, though weekly innings limits have been in use for decades in youth baseball. In theory, pitch limits would improve safety.	Moderate
Pitch types [25, 26, 57]	There is no evidence that prohibiting pitch types that young pitchers use reduces the risk of arm injury. In theory this may improve safety, but no studies have been conducted.	Fair

helped develop these helmets and disseminate this information throughout organized baseball [56]. While head and facial injuries still occur to batters, they are much less frequent than they would be without batting helmets.

Research has demonstrated a reduction in the risk of facial and eye injuries with the use of face guards while batting [12, 35]. Marshall et al. [12] found an approximately 35% reduction in risk of facial injury in youth leagues using face shields compared to youth leagues without. Face shields are currently used in virtually all younger youth baseball leagues and many older youth baseball leagues. High school players have not consistently used face shields, likely because the ability to see high velocity pitches and breaking pitches is compromised even with a clear plastic visor. This balance between safety and performance is one made almost daily by athletes in all sports at all levels. Given that younger players are at higher risk of injury from pitched or batted balls [10, 29, 36], this shift from face shield use to non-use represents a shift in the balance between safety and performance.

Safety Baseballs

Several companies have developed a variety of low-impact baseballs for use by youth baseball leagues to reduce the likelihood of injury from blunt impact trauma from a thrown or batted ball [12, 44]. These balls are designed to mimic the play characteristics of a regulation hard ball, but with softer materials. Some laboratory testing suggests that these balls may increase the risk of ocular trauma because the ball deforms deeper into the eye socket, causing more damage to eye tissue [45]. However, the large number of other injuries that may be prevented including fractures and *commotio cordis* may justify the potential increased risk of serious ocular trauma, particularly if these balls are used in conjunction with face shields. A recent study by Marshall et al. [12] evaluated the risk of injury in leagues using softer baseballs and found an approximately 23% reduction in risk of ball-related injury.

Breakaway Bases

While research has been conducted in proper sliding techniques [46, 47], breakaway bases likely provide a much greater risk reduction without a substantial increase in cost (current designs cost approximately what traditional bases do) [47]. The increased safety achieved with these breakaway base designs appears unequivocal and should be used to reduce serious slide-related sprains and fractures seen at all levels of play [47, 58].

Proper Techniques

Many coaches, baseball experts, and researchers claim to know the best or safest way to perform baseball skills such as pitching, hitting, fielding, or baserunning, but there is currently a paucity of scientific evidence that any of these techniques are meaningfully safer or result in improved performance.

Pitching Limits

Youth baseball leagues regulate the number of innings pitchers pitch per week, but the current standards may be inadequate to prevent arm injuries. Unfortunately, no systematic research on the effect of these changes was undertaken and studies from before and after the intervention are not readily comparable due to differences in the measurement of injury and broader societal changes that may influence changes in injury risk.

Youth leagues currently have limits on the number of innings pitched (e.g. 6–12 innings pitched per week) and required rest periods (e.g. minimum of 48 hours rest after at least two innings pitched). These regulations apply to all pitchers within a youth league organization [59]. A difficulty with this regulatory system is that younger pitchers tend to throw more pitches per inning than older pitchers because they have less control over their pitches because of lack of experience, greater musculoskeletal immaturity, or both [60]. Therefore, with innings limits, those with potentially weaker and less developed arms are throwing more pitches than those with stronger arms. It is possible that these youth league organizations could more effectively prevent these injuries in pitchers with pitch limits or batter limits. To educate about the potential safety benefits of pitch count limits, the Medical and Safety Committee of USA Baseball published a position statement on their website (www.usabaseball.com/ med_position_statement.html).

Pitch Types

Curveballs and other breaking pitches have long been implicated anecdotally with arm injuries in children, but until recently, the association has not been scientifically established [25, 26]. While evidence now suggests that the risk of arm problems is elevated with breaking pitch use, it may not be strong enough to discourage children, parents, and coaches from using breaking pitches, because breaking pitches provide a distinct advantage against young batters.

Perhaps a more compelling argument against the use of breaking pitches among young pitchers is based upon the childhood dream of becoming a major league baseball player. Dr. Joe Chandler of the Atlanta Braves explained that this team was much more interested in pitching velocity, pitch location, and the ability to change speeds (i.e. throw a change-up) than in the ability to throw breaking pitches [57]. In fact, the average age at which pitchers in the Atlanta Braves organization learned to throw a curveball was 14.5 years. Therefore, there may be long-term benefits for a youth pitcher to concentrate on arm strength for velocity, accuracy for pitch location, and getting batters out with a strong fastball and slow change-up rather than relying on curveballs to get batters out more easily.

Suggestions for Future Research

The primary challenges in sports injury prevention research in general and baseball injury prevention research in particular, is the definition of 'injury' and the definition of 'exposure'. The studies reviewed here used a variety of injury definitions from self-reported pain to an injury requiring missed games or practices to emergency room care to insurance claims. A clear and consistent definition of injury is vital to additional and improved understanding of baseball injuries.

Furthermore, exposure has been defined in a variety of ways from counting players to counting games or practices to counting pitches. Given that many of the current sports injury surveillance systems use a measure of athlete-exposures (one athlete exposure is one game or practice session for one athlete), this is probably the best definition of exposure and allows for future studies to be compared with many previous studies in the literature. However, this is really only an acceptable exposure definition of non-pitchers. Starting pitchers and relief pitchers have very different exposure levels during a pitching appearance so number of innings, batters, or pitches may be a better marker of exposure.

Future research efforts should focus primarily on identifying safe pitching mechanics for young pitchers and identifying the optimal balance point between skill development and safety in pitchers – the balance between pitching too much and too little. With the proven effectiveness of safety baseballs, face shields, and breakaway bases, the next wave of equipment innovation should focus on making a face shield that is acceptable to players at higher skill levels, developing a soft baseball that has play characteristics identical to traditional baseballs, and identifying other equipment improvements that can protect young baseball players as they enjoy the game.

These research endeavors would ideally be conducted using randomized controlled intervention trial methodology unless impractical. In those cases, the research should be conducted using a prospective cohort design.

References

1   USA Baseball. This is USA Baseball. internet. 2004.
2   American Academy of Pediatrics: Risk of injury from baseball and softball in children. Pediatrics 2001;107:782–784.
3   Pasternack JS, Veenema KR, Callahan CM: Baseball injuries: A Little League survey. Pediatrics 1996;98:445–448.
4   Walter S, Hart L: Application of epidemiological methodology to sports and exercise science research; in Pandolf K, Holloszy J (eds): Exercise and Sports Science Reviews, ed1. Baltimore, Williams & Wilkens, 1990, pp 417–448.
5   Chambers RB: Orthopaedic injuries in athletes (ages 6 to 17). Comparison of injuries occurring in six sports. Am J Sports Med 1979;7:195–197.
6   Cheng TL, Fields CB, Brenner RA, Wright JL, Lomax T, Scheidt PC: Sports injuries: An important cause of morbidity in urban youth. District of Columbia Child/Adolescent Injury Research Network. Pediatrics 2000;105:E32.
7   DuRant RH, Pendergrast RA, Seymore C, Gaillard G, Donner J: Findings from the preparticipation athletic examination and athletic injuries. Am J Dis Child 1992;146:85–91.
8   Garrick JG, Requa RK: Injuries in high school sports. Pediatrics 1978;61:465–469.

9   Grana WA: Summary of 1978–79 injury registry for Oklahoma secondary schools. J Oklahoma Med Assoc 1979;72:369–372.

10   Hale CJ: Injuries among 771,810 little league baseball players. J Sports Med Phys Fitness 1961;1:80–83.

11   Lowe EB, Perkins ER, Herndon JH: Rhode Island high school athletic injuries 1985–1986. RI Med J 1987;70:265–270.

12   Marshall SW, Mueller FO, Kirby DP, Yang J: Evaluation of safety balls and faceguards for prevention of injuries in youth baseball. JAMA 2003;289:568–574.

13   Martin RK, Yesalis CE, Foster D, Albright JP: Sports injuries at the 1985 Junior Olympics. Am J Sports Med 1987;15:603–608.

14   McClain LG, Reynolds S: Sports injuries in high school. Pediatrics 1989;84:446–450.

15   Powell JW, Barber-Foss KD: Sex-related injury patterns among selected high school sports. Am J Sports Med 2000;28:385–391.

16   Radelet MA, Lephart SM, Rubinstein EN, Myers JB: Survey of the injury rate for children in community sports. Pediatrics 2002;110:e28.

17   Zaricznyj B, Shattuck LJM, Mast TA, Roberston RV, Delia G: Sports-related injuries in school age children. Am J Sports Med 1980;8:318–324.

18   Francis R, Bunch T, Chandler B: Little league elbow: A decade later. Phys Sportsmed 1978;6:88–94.

19   Adams JE: Injury to the throwing arm: A study of traumatic changes in the elbow joints of boy baseball players. Calif Med 1965;102:127–132.

20   Albright JA, Jokl P, Shaw R, Albright JP: Clinical study of baseball pitchers: Correlation of injury to the throwing arm with method of delivery. Am J Sports Med 1978;6:15–21.

21   Grana WA, Rashkin A: Pitcher's elbow in adolescents. Am J Sports Med 1980;8:333–336.

22   Gugenheim JJ Jr, Stanley RF, Woods GW, Tullos HS: Little League survey: The Houston study. Am J Sports Med 1976;4:189–200.

23   Hang YS, Lippert FG III, Spolek GA, Frankel VH, Harrington RM: Biomechanical study of the pitching elbow. Int Orthop 1979;3:217–223.

24   Larson RL, Singer KM, Bergstrom R, Thomas S: Little League survey: The Eugene study. Am J Sports Med 1976;4:201–209.

25   Lyman S, Fleisig GS, Waterbor JW, Funkhouser EM, Pulley L, Andrews JR, Osinski ED, Roseman JM: Longitudinal study of elbow and shoulder pain in youth baseball pitchers. Med Sci Sports Exerc 2001;33:1803–1810.

26   Lyman S, Fleisig GS, Andrews JR, Osinski ED: Effect of pitch type, pitch count, and pitching mechanics on risk of elbow and shoulder pain in youth baseball pitchers. Am J Sports Med 2002;30:463–468.

27   Ochi, T, Shimaoka Y, Nakagawa S: Enactment of a provision for restricting pitching in national high school championship games. Clin Sports Med 1994;11:851–853.

28   Torg JS, Pollack H, Sweterlitsch P: The effect of competitive pitching on the shoulders and elbows of preadolescent baseball players. Pediatrics 1972;49:267–272.

29   Hale CJ: Protective Equipment for Baseball. Phys Sportsmed 1979;7:58–63.

30   Andrews JR, Fleisig GS: Preventing throwing injuries. J Orthop Sports Phys Ther 1998;27:187–188.

31   Yen KL, Metzl JD: Sports-specific concerns in the young athlete: Baseball. Pediatr Emerg Care 2000;16:215–220.

32   Carson WG Jr, Gasser SI: Little Leaguer's shoulder. A report of 23 cases. Am J Sports Med 1998;26:575–580.

33   Janda DH, Wojtys EM, Hankin FM, Benedict ME: Softball sliding injuries. A prospective study comparing standard and modified bases. JAMA 1988;259:1848–1850.

34   Danis RP, Hu K, Bell M: Acceptability of baseball face guards and reduction of oculofacial injury in receptive youth league players. Inj Prev 2000;6:232–234.

35   Powell JW, Barber-Foss KD: Traumatic brain injury in high school athletes. JAMA 1999;282:958–963.

36   Heald J: Summary of baseball/softball injuries. 1991. Tullahoma, TN, Worth Sports Company. Ref Type: Pamphlet.

37   Hutchinson MR, Ireland ML: Overuse and throwing injuries in the skeletally immature athlete. Instr Course Lect 2003;52:25–36.

38 Hale CJ: Little Leaguer's shoulder: A report of 23 cases. Am J Sports Med 1999;27:269.

39 Lipscomb AB: Baseball pitching injuries in growing athletes. J Sports Med 1975;3:25–34.

40 Hennigan SP, Bush-Joseph CA, Kuo KN, Bach BR Jr: Throwing-induced humeral shaft fracture in skeletally immature adolescents. Orthopedics 1999;22:621–622.

41 Abrunzo TJ: Commotio cordis. The single, most common cause of traumatic death in youth baseball. Am J Dis Child 1991;145:1279–1282.

42 Maron BJ, Poliac LC, Kaplan JA, Mueller FO: Blunt impact to the chest leading to sudden death from cardiac arrest during sports activities. N Engl J Med 1995;333:337–342.

43 Maron BJ, Gohman TE, Kyle SB, Estes NA III, Link MS: Clinical profile and spectrum of commotio cordis. JAMA 2002;287:1142–1146.

44 Yamamoto LG, Inaba AS, Okamura DM, Yamamoto JA, Yamamoto JB: Injury reduction and bounce characteristics of safety baseballs and acceptability by youth leagues. Clin Pediatr (Phila) 2001;40:197–203.

45 Vinger PF, Duma SM, Crandall J: Baseball hardness as a risk factor for eye injuries. Arch Ophthalmol 1999;117:354–358.

46 Janda DH, Bir C, Kedroske B: A comparison of standard vs. breakaway bases: An analysis of a preventative intervention for softball and baseball foot and ankle injuries. Foot Ankle Int 2001;22: 810–816.

47 Sendre RA, Keating TM, Hornak JE, Newitt PA: Use of the Hollywood Impact Base and standard stationary base to reduce sliding and base-running injuries in baseball and softball. Am J Sports Med 1994;22:450–453.

48 Fleisig GS, Andrews JR, Dillman CJ, Escamilla RF: Kinetics of baseball pitching with implications about injury mechanisms. Am J Sports Med 1995;23:233–239.

49 Fleisig GS, Barrentine SW, Escamilla RF, Andrews JR: Biomechanics of overhand throwing with implications for injuries. Sports Med 1996;21:421–437.

50 Dillman CJ, Fleisig GS, Andrews JR: Biomechanics of pitching with emphasis upon shoulder kinematics. J Orthop Sports Phys Ther 1993;18:402–408.

51 Fleisig GS, Dillman CJ, Andrews JR: Proper mechanics for baseball pitching. Clin Sports Med 1989;1:151–170.

52 Fleisig GS: The biomechanics of baseball pitching; Thesis, University of Alabama at Birmingham, 1994.

53 Fleisig GS, Barrentine SW, Zheng N, Escamilla RF, Andrews JR: Kinematic and kinetic comparison of baseball pitching among various levels of development. J Biomech 1999;32:1371–1375.

54 Elliott B, Grove JR, Gibson B, Thurston B: Three-dimensional cinematographic analysis of the fastball and curveball pitches in baseball. Int J Sport Biomech 1986;2:20–28.

55 Escamilla RF, Fleisig GS, Barrentine SW, Zheng N, Andrews JR: Kinematic comparisons of throwing different types of baseball pitches. J Appl Biomech 1998;14:1–23.

56 Hale CJ, Lyman S, Fleisig GS: 1998. Pers. Commun.

57 Chandler J: The epidemic of baseball injuries in youth baseball – Is prevention possible? Birmingham AL, American Sports Medicine Institute. Proceedings of the 21st Annual Injuries in Baseball Course. 1–23–2003.

58 Janda DH, Hankin FM, Wojtys EM: Softball injuries: Cost, cause and prevention. Am Fam Physician 1986;33:143–144.

59 Andrews JR, Fleisig GS: Medical and Safety Advisory Committee Special Report: How many pitches should I allow my child to throw? USA Baseball News 5, 1996.

60 Axe MJ, Snyder-Mackler L, Konin JG, Strube MJ: Development of a distance-based interval throwing program for Little League-aged athletes. Am J Sports Med 1996;24:594–602.

Dr. Stephen Lyman
Hospital for Special Surgery
Forster Center for Clinical Outcome Research
535 E. 70th Street, New York, NY 10021 (USA)
Tel. +1 212 774 7125, Fax +1 212 774 2455, E-Mail lymans@hss.edu

Maffulli N, Caine DJ (eds): Epidemiology of Pediatric Sports Injuries: Team Sports.
Med Sport Sci. Basel, Karger, 2005, vol 49, pp 31–61

······················

Basketball Injuries

Peter A. Harmer

Exercise Science-Sports Medicine, Willamette University, Salem, Oreg., USA

Abstract

Objective: To identify and quantify, to the best extent possible from the existing
literature, injury characteristics and factors (risk; protective) associated with injury in young
basketball players. **Data Sources:** Database searches principally involving Medline and
SportDiscus. In addition, web-based searching and filtering of the reference lists of papers
found in the preliminary searches were utilized. **Main Results:** Few well-controlled studies
of this population have been conducted. However, from the information available: basketball
is the most frequent cause of sports-related emergency department visits for youth and
adolescents; the risk of being injured in a game is greater than for practice; girls are more
likely to be injured than boys, especially with knee and ankle injuries and the knee injuries are
more likely to be severe; acute injuries are more common than chronic; strains/sprains are the
most common types of injuries but overall time loss is minimal, indicating that the majority
of pediatric basketball injuries are minor (less than 7 days away from activity). Intervention
studies show that: mouthguards reduce orofacial/dental injuries; mouthguard use can be
increased in young players; neuromuscular training can reduce the incidence of knee injuries
in female participants; postural sway is related to risk of ankle injury. **Conclusions:** The current state of epidemiological research involving youth and adolescent basketball injuries is
poor. With an increasing number of young participants, in situations ranging from informal
play and physical education classes to organized community and school teams, the need for
comprehensive and authoritative information on risk and protective factors is significant.

Copyright © 2005 S. Karger AG, Basel

Introduction

Basketball is one of the most popular physical activities in the world: 11%
of the world plays basketball and the Fédération Internationale de Basketball
(FIBA), the international governing body of basketball, now represents 212
member nations and 450 million registered participants [1]. In the USA, basketball is the most popular team sport for boys and girls, with 544,811 boys and

457,986 girls registered in the 2003–2004 school year [2]. Although the USA has long been considered the dominant force in basketball, recent results such as in the men's 1988 and 2004 Olympic Games and 2002 World Championships demonstrate that the rest of the world is closing the gap. The evolving parity at the upper echelon of the sport is only possible with the on-going growth of developmental programs for children and youth. Similarly, since the first women's world championship in 1953, many countries are providing opportunities for youngsters to learn the game in settings ranging from physical education classes and scholastic competition to governmental and private sports organizations and community recreational programs.

Unfortunately, as the number of young male and female participants has increased so has the number of injuries. For example, according to the National Electronic Injury Surveillance System – All Injury Program (NEISS-AIP) [3], basketball was the most common cause of sports- and recreation-related injuries seen at USA Emergency Departments in 2000–2001, with 395,251 cases. The proportion of cases was not evenly distributed across age groups – for boys aged 5–9, basketball accounted for 4.9% of all sport injuries, whereas it constituted 15.2% of cases for boys aged 10–14, and 25.9% for boys aged 15–19, the highest percentage for any activity in this group including football. For girls aged 10–14, basketball produced 14.9% of all sports injuries and 18.1% in the 15–19-year-old group.

Although the absolute number of injuries has implications for the healthcare system, the actual risk of injury in basketball is difficult to determine. The apparent age-related increases in injury in the NEISS-AIP may be simply a reflection of the number of players at each age level. Without knowing the number of participants, it is not possible to determine whether older children are more at risk and, if so, why. Similarly, even accurately identifying the extent of the problem is difficult. If NEISS data from physician offices and urgent-care clinics are incorporated, the number of basketball injuries in 5–14 year olds was estimated to be approximately 574,000 [4]. In either case, these data represent only 20–50% of the actual number of basketball injuries in participants aged under 18 [3, 5].

If effective interventions are to be instituted to reduce injuries in young players, accurate and reliable information is essential. However, the limited epidemiological data available center on college and professional athletes, although participation is much greater in scholastic competition [6]. Zvijac and Thompson [6] proposed that studying high school players would provide a clear understanding of the true nature of injuries in basketball because more data could be obtained from the larger population. Although this approach is reasonable, it assumes that etiological factors are static across the wide variety of player and playing characteristics, but both direct and indirect evidence indicates this is not the case. Physical, psychological, and social traits of five year olds are significantly different from those of 18 year olds, as are the demands of playing in physical education class, pick-up games, or organized competition in the Americas, Europe, Asia or Australia. Data from the appropriate stratification of gender, age, environment, and sociocultural factors are necessary to uncover, and effectively counter, the underlying risks of playing basketball.

This review identifies and evaluates the available literature on injuries in pediatric basketball. The primary search was limited to data-based studies in English derived from the Medline and SportDiscus databases, utilizing combinations of both general ('basketball', 'injury', 'youth, pediatric, children'), and specific terms ('catastrophic', 'eye', 'dental'). Secondary searching consisted of combing the reference lists of acceptable studies from the primary search and a previous review on basketball injuries [6], as well as a general web-based search using the same keywords.

Results demonstrated an overall lack of quality information for pediatric basketball injuries. A large number of hospital emergency department-based studies provided a general picture of the relative public health burden of basketball injuries but did not provide stratified age, injury type, location or severity data. For example, Watkins and Peabody [7] completed a 3-year retrospective study of sports injuries in athletes aged 5–17 treated at a sports injury clinic in London and found that, for males, basketball was eighth on a list of 10 sports ranked by the number of injuries reported, accounting for only 3.7% of injuries, while Boyce and Quigley [8] reported that basketball accounted for 7% of sports-related injuries in 5–16 year olds at a Scottish Emergency Department over a 3-month period.

However, in a similar study in Hong Kong over a 6-year period, basketball accounted for 15.5% (37 of 238 cases) of all sports-related injuries in children younger than 16 years old, the most of any sport [9], as was the finding from a 6-year study at the national Olympic Training Center in Puerto Rico for athletes 10–19 years old [10]. Unfortunately, none of these studies presented exposure information; so it is impossible to determine whether the differences were due to the popularity of basketball in each location, or whether there is a causal mechanism operating that makes playing basketball 'riskier' in Hong Kong and Puerto Rico than in England or Scotland.

Methodological problems in hospital-based studies, include: (1) focus is often not on specific sports, (2) lack of a universal definition of injury making comparison across studies difficult, (3) no distinction between formal and recreational activities, (4) no denominator data (reference population), and (5) the metric for incidence rates is not standardized. In the majority of these, and similar school- or club-based studies, basketball-specific information about age, gender, and injury characteristics is inextricably embedded in broader analytical categories [11]. In addition, many references are out-dated as the nature of basketball has changed (from noncontact to contact), and younger age groups are generally not included [12].

Given the impact of basketball across the globe, the dearth of methodologically sound injury research on young players is surprising. If suitable preventative and protective measures are to evolve, future work needs to include a clear understanding of the population at risk, definitive criteria for a reportable injury, and the capacity to calculate exposure time and time loss.

Incidence of Injury

Delineating the risk of injury in sport is based on establishing the incidence, i.e., the number of new cases that occur in a particular population over a given time. Although the number of cases alone can be informative [13], incidence is considered the gold standard of the measure of risk. A comparison of injury rates from prospective and retrospective research is shown in table 1 and covers high school [14–21], physical education class [22], clubs/sports organizations [23–27], and hospital emergency departments [28, 29]. In addition, studies reporting incidence data specifically for knee [18, 19, 30], ankle [31, 32], head [33], and orofacial [34–36] injuries are listed. Unfortunately, the injury literature on youth basketball suffers from a broad range of methodological shortcomings, including widely varying definitions of a reportable injury, limited measures of exposure, differing metrics of risk, and poor delineation of the population at risk. Consequently, it is very difficult to get a clear picture of the risk inherent in basketball, or the particular risks associated with gender, age, level of skill, playing conditions, etc. Although some studies have been well designed, the lack of a coordinated research program has produced a somewhat fragmented picture from which only broad conclusions may be drawn.

For example, the 1997–1998 National Hospital Ambulatory Medical Care Survey (NHAMCS) of emergency department admissions for ages 5–24 (40% aged 5–14) showed that basketball was the most frequently cited reason for sport-related emergency department visits (17.1%), with a calculated incidence rate of 5.8 per 1,000 (95% CI = 4.7–6.8) persons in the general population [37]. Although the 1997–1999 National Health Interview Survey (NHIS) had a 36.2% difference in the number of reported basketball injuries with NHAMCS, it confirmed basketball as the most common cause of sports injury for ages 5–24, with a rate of 3.9 per 1,000 persons (95% CI = 3.3–4.5) in the general population. However, for the group ages 5–14, basketball had an incidence rate of 6.5 per 1,000 persons (95% CI = 4.7–8.3) [38]. NHIS also found that 42%

Table 1. A comparison of injury rates among young basketball players

Study	Design Prospective/ Retrospective (P) (R)	Data collection Direct monitor (DM), Interview (I), Record review (RR), Questionnaire (Q)	Duration of study	Team type	Number of injuries (definition varies greatly)	Number of participants	Injury rate per 100 participants	Injury rate per 1,000 hours of exposure	Injury rate per 1,000 AE
Chandy and Grana [14]	?	RR	3 years (1978–1981)	High school (n = 130) (USA)	404 (boys) 498 (girls)	7,209 (boys) 6,426 (girls)	5.6 7.8	– –	– –
McLain and Reynolds [15]	P	DM	1 year (1987–1988)	High school (n = 1) (USA)	21 (boys) 14 (girls)	57 (boys) 45 (girls)	36.8 31.0	– –	– –
DuRant et al. [16]	R	Q	1 year (1989–1990)	High school (n = multiple) (USA)	20 (boys) 32 (girls)	132 (boys) 96 (girls)	15.2 33.3	– –	– –
Gomez et al. [17]	P	DM	1 year (1993–1994)	High school (n = 100) (USA)	436	890 (girls)	49	4	–
Messina et al. [18]	P	DM	1 season (1996–1997)	High school (n = 100) (USA)	543 436	973 (boys) 890 (girls)	– –	3.2 3.6	– –
Powell and Barber-Foss [19]	P	DM	3 years (1995–1997)	High school (n = 246) (USA)	1,933 (boys) 1,748 (girls)	6,831 (boys) 6,083 (girls)	28.3 (boys) 28.7 (girls)	– –	– –
Beachy et al. [20]	P	DM	8 years (1988–1995)	High school private (USA)	505 (boys) 467 (girls)	541 (boys) 587 (girls)	93 80	– –	– –
Weir and Watson [21]	R	Q	1 year (?Mid-1990s?)	High school (IRL)	22	?	–	5.6	–
Beckx et al. [22]	P	DM;RR	7 months (1982–1983)	PE classes/club (ages 8–16) (NED)	–	Mixed activity population	99.8*	<5 (practice) 23 (game)	–

Table 1 (continued)

Study	Design Prospective/ Retrospective (P) (R)	Data Collection Direct monitor (DM), Interview (I), Record review (RR), Questionnaire (Q)	Duration of study	Team type	Number of injuries (definition varies greatly)	Number of participants	Injury rate per 100 participants	Injury rate per 1,000 hours of exposure	Injury rate per 1,000 AE
Gutgesell [23]	P	DM	1 season (1989–1990)	YMCA (ages 5–12) (USA)	25 (boys) / 14 (girls)	406 (boys) / 104 (girls)	6.16 / 13.46	– / –	4.86 (combined)
Chambers [24]	P	DM	1 year (1976–1977)	Military base (ages 6–17) (USA)	4**	625	–	0.88	–
Yde and Nielsen [25]	P	DM;I;Q	1 season (1985–1986)	Sports club (DEN)	21	52 (boys: 27; girls: 29)	–	3	–
de Loës [26]	R	RR	3 years (1987–1989)	National organization (ages 14–20) (SUI)	243 (boys) / 229 (female)	15,094 (boys) / 10,154 (girls)	–	0.35 / 0.49	– / –
Hickey et al. [27]	R	RR	6 years (1990–1995)	Sport institute (ages 16–18) (AUS)	223	49 (girls)	290*	–	–
Prebble et al. [28]	R	RR	6 years (1988–1994)	Rural ED (USA)	1,210[a] / 782[b]	1,010[a] / 629[b]	119.8[a] / 80.4[b]	– / –	– / –
Damore et al. [29]	R	RR	2 months (1999–2000)	Hospital ED (4) (Mean age 12) (USA)	111	94 (male patients) / 14 (female patients)	–	–	–

Specific location studies
Knee only

Study	Design Prospective/ Retrospective (P) (R)	Data Collection Direct monitor (DM), Interview (I), Record review (RR), Questionnaire (Q)	Duration of study	Team type	Number of injuries (definition varies greatly)	Number of participants	Injury rate per 100 participants	Injury rate per 1,000 hours of exposure	Injury rate per 1,000 AE
Messina et al. [18]	P	DM	1 season (1996–1997)	High school (n = 100) (USA)	53 (boys) / 86 (girls)	– / –	– / –	0.31 / 0.71	– / –

Study			Setting	Period	No. injured	No. participants			
Powell and Barber-Foss [19]	P	DM	High school (n = 246) (USA)	3 years (1995–1997)	251 (boys) / 275 (girls)	6,831 (boys) / 6,083 (girls)	3.7 / 4.5	– / –	– / –
de Loës et al. [30]	R	RR	National organization (ages 14–20) (SUI)	7 years (1987–1993)	68 (boys) / 78 (girls)	– / –	– / –	0.04 / 0.06	– / –
Ankle only									
McGuine et al. [31]	P	DM	High school (n = 5) (USA)	2 seasons (1997–1999)	– / –	119 (boys)[c] / 91 (girls)[c]	– / –	– / –	1.68 / 1.44
Hosea et al. [32]	P	DM	High school (n = 125) (USA)	2 years (?Mid-1990s?)	480 (boys) / 424 (girls)	6,336 (boys) / 4,576 (girls)	7.5 / 9.2	– / –	– / –
Head and face only									
Powell and Barber-Foss [33] (MTBI only)	P	DM	High school (n = 235) (USA)	3 years (1995–1997)	51[d] / 63[d]	6,831 (boys) / 6,083 (girls)	– / –	– / –	0.11 / 0.16
Maestrello-deMoya and Primosch [34] (orofacial only)	R	Q	High school (n = 3) (USA)	1 year (1986–1987)	315	1,020	30.9		
Kvittem et al. [35] (orofacial only)	P	DM	High school (n = 7) (USA)	1 year (1996–1997)	56	101	56.3	–	
Teo et al. [36] (dental only)	R	Q	High school (SIN)	Ever injured (?Mid-1990s?)	30	154 (boys)	19	–	

*per 100 participants per year – very broad definition of injury.
**Significant orthopedic injuries only.
[a] Includes 12.1% aged 20–29.
[b] Aged <19 years old.
[c] Specifically selected group for prevention study (asymptomatic, no time loss ankle or knee injuries for 12 months).
[d] Reportable if evaluated.

of this age group did not attend an emergency department for treatment. Nonetheless, the two studies provide some framework for understanding the injury characteristics for young basketball players. Additionally, Kelm et al. [39] reported that basketball accounted for 19.6% of injuries in physical education classes in Germany in children 11–15 years old, and studies from Dutch and Swiss schools indicated that basketball has a relative risk of 1.3 (95% CI = 1.2–1.4) to 1.99 compared to the mean rate of all sports injuries recorded [11, 40].

The data in table 1 highlight the difficulty of gaining an accurate impression of the risks in youth basketball. Definitions of reportable injury range from any incident evaluated to incidents that result in at least 2 days absence, and the metric of risk include percentage injured, injuries per 1,000 hours of exposure or per 1,000 athlete exposures. Moreover, with the variety of ages in disparate settings (school teams, clubs, physical education classes) across multiple countries, there is little appropriately comparable data. Even the results of the most commonly studied population (American public high school players) vary considerably, from 5.6–36.8 per 100 participants for boys, and 7.8–49 per 100 participants for girls [14–17, 19], although two studies which report injuries per 1,000 hours of participation are similar (3.2–4.0) [17, 18]. A coordinated research program with standard protocols is necessary if a clear picture of the level of risk, and associated causal factors, is to emerge.

Injury Characteristics

Injury Onset

There are few data available to determine the relative risk of sustaining an acute versus a chronic injury in youth basketball. However, two studies with significantly differing populations support the proposition of a greater risk of acute injury. Weir and Watson [21] found a relative risk of acute to chronic injury of 2.5:1 in a one year study of Irish high schools students (average age 14 years, with 4.02 acute injures per 1,000 h of participation vs. 1.61 chronic injuries per 1,000 h participation). Similarly, a 6 year study of elite females (average age 17 years) at a national training center in Australia evidenced an average acute-chronic injury ratio of 1.66:1 (range 0.88:1–2.9:1) [27].

Injury Location

A percent comparison of injury location in youth basketball is shown in table 2 [12, 17–19, 25, 27, 29, 41–43]. The lower extremities generally account for the majority of injuries in youth basketball (35.9–92%), with the ankle/foot representing the single most frequently injured region (16.6–44%) [12, 17–19,

Table 2. A percent comparison of injury location in youth basketball

Location	Taylor and Attia [12] (n = 132)	Gomez et al. [17] (n = 890)	Messina et al. [18] boys (n = 543)	girls (n = 436)	Powell and Barber-Foss [19] boys (n = 1,933)	girls (n = 1,748)	Yde and Nielsen [25] (n = 21)	Hickey et al. [27] (n = 223)	Damore et al. [29] (n = 111)
Head/Spine/ Trunk	(11.4)	(14)	(20)	(14)	(21.3)	(18.7)	–	(20.7)	(7)
Skull	10.7 (including face)	3	3	3	–	–	–	5.8 (including face)	2
Face		4	11	5	10 (including scalp)	6.8	–		3
Teeth	–	–	–	–	–	–	–	–	–
Neck	–	–	–	–	–	–	–	–	–
Back	–	6	5	6	–	–	–	14.9	2
Upper extremity	(48.9)	(15)	(16)	(14)	(13.8)	(12.8)	(43)	(13.0)	(35)
Shoulder	1.5	5	4	3	2.4	2.4	–	3.1 (including arm/elbow)	1
Arm	–	–	–	–	–	–	–		–
Elbow	–	–	–	–	–	–	–	–	–
Forearm	–	–	–	–	11.4	10.4	–	–	13
Wrist	36.7 (including hand)	2	3	3	(including wrist/hand)		–	9.9 (including hand)	(including wrist)
Hand/ Fingers		8	9	8	–	–	43		21

Table 2 (continued)

Location	Taylor and Attia [12] (n = 132)	Gomez et al. [17] (n = 890)	Messina et al. [18] boys (n = 543)	girls (n = 436)	Powell and Barber-Foss [19] boys (n = 1,933)	girls (n = 1,748)	Yde and Nielsen [25] (n = 21)	Hickey et al. [27] (n = 223)	Damore et al. [29] (n = 111)
Lower extremity	(37.1)	(69)	(61)	(69)	(64.8)	(68.7)	(43)	(62.4)	(58)
Pelvis/Hips	–	10	11	9	–	–	–	6.3	–
Thigh	–	(including thigh)	(including thigh)		–	–	5	(including thigh)	1
Knee	–	19	10	20	11.1	15.7	5	18.8	7
Leg	–	4	4	4	–	–	–	10.8	6
Ankle	33.3	31	32	31	39.3	36.6	33	16.6	44
Foot/Toes	(including foot)	5	4	5	(including foot)		–	9.9	(including foot)
	2.7% other	2% not listed	(3% other)				14% other	4% chest	

Location	NATA [41] 1986–1988 boys	girls	1995–1997 boys	girls	Belechri et al. [42] DEN	FRA	GRE	NED	UK	Finch et al. [43] (n = 3,722)
Head/Spine/ Trunk	–	–	(12.2)	(8.8)	(4.6)	(5.2)	(8.8)	(6)	(8.2)	(14.4)
Skull	–	–	–	–	–	–	–	–	–	–
Face	–	–	12.2	8.8	2.7	3.1	6.2	4	6.3	–

Body location									
Teeth	—	—	(and scalp)	—	—	—	—	—	—
Neck	—	—	—	—	—	—	—	—	—
Back	—	—	—	—	—	—	—	—	—
Upper extremity	(92)	—	(63.3)	(71.1)	(71)	(67.5)	(69)	(72)	(58.5)
Shoulder	—	—	—	—	—	—	—	—	—
Arm	—	—	—	7.7	19.5	27.3	20	21.2	—
Elbow	—	—	—	—	—	—	—	—	—
Forearm	—	—	11.5	—	—	—	—	—	—
Wrist	—	—	11.2 (and wrist/hand)	—	—	—	—	—	—
Hand/ Fingers	—	—	—	63.4	51.5	40.2	49	50.8	—
Lower extremity	(50)	—	(65.6)	(24.3)	(23.8)	(23.7)	(26)	(19.8)	(25.1)
Pelvis/ Hips	—	—	−4.7	—	—	—	—	—	—
Thigh	11	—	16.6 (and thigh/leg)	—	—	—	—	—	—
Knee	9	18	−0.3 13	4.8	6.2	4.1	5	7.7	—
Leg	—	—	—	—	—	—	—	—	—
Ankle	42	32	38.3 36	14.4	14.5	15.2	14	8.2	—
Foot/Toes	(and foot)	(and foot)	—	—	—	—	—	—	—

23, 25, 27–29, 41]. The knee is the second most frequently injured area in the lower extremity (5–20%) [17–19, 25, 27, 29, 41] but with noticeable gender differences, ranging from 9–11.1% for boys to 13–20% for girls [18, 19, 41]. In a stark comparison, Belechri et al. [42], reporting data from five European Union countries, indicated a range for total lower extremities injuries of 19.8–26%, with ankle/foot injuries contributing just 8.2–15.2% of all injuries, and knee injuries ranging from 4.1–7.7% of the total. An Australian study similarly reported lower extremity injuries accounting for only 25.1% [43].

The reversal of findings is repeated in upper extremities data with most studies reporting between 11–16% [17–19, 27, 41] or 35–49% [12, 25, 29] of injuries occurring in this region in contrast to Belechri et al. [42] with values from 67.5–72% and Finch et al. [43] at 58.5%. The majority of upper extremities injuries in Belechri et al.'s [42] study were to the hand/fingers (40.2–63.4%), in line with additional studies, particularly involving younger children (13% [23]; 13.7% of acute injuries [27]; 17% [44]; 19.3% [28]; 21% [29]; 43% [25]). Taylor and Attia [12] found that wrist/hand injuries were more likely in basketball than in any other sport studied (OR = 1.7; 95% CI = 1.1–2.5). However, the reason for the extreme deviation of the European and Australian data is not evident.

The percentage of injuries to other body areas, particularly the head, varies between 7–21%. Head injuries producing mild traumatic brain injury (MTBI) have been found to account for approximately 2.6 and 3.6% of all basketball injuries in males and females, respectively [33]. Face and mouth injuries vary between 3–12.2% of all injuries [12, 18, 27, 29, 41] with the nose (epistaxis in 12.8% of all injuries [23]) and teeth apparently the most vulnerable [17, 35, 45, 46]. Finally, Wan et al. [47] reported that, from data in the National Pediatric Trauma Registry (1990–1999), basketball accounted for 9.4% of significant abdominal injuries (18 of 191 cases) reported in 5–18 year olds. The kidneys and spleen were most at risk [5 cases (28%) each]. There was one liver injury and the other 7 were nonspecific abdominal injuries.

Situational

The risk of injury is significantly greater in games than in practice. Estimates vary greatly, depending on the characteristics of the study. For example, in a study of children aged 5–12 in a community program, 90% of injuries were game-related, with a relative risk of 16.9:1 [23]. However, 6–18 year olds in a Danish sports club showed a game:practice relative risk of 2.4:1 (games = 5.7 injuries per 1,000 h of participation; practice = 2.4) [25]. Two studies of high school players in the USA produced a relative risk of 6.8:1 for female players in a 100-school sample [17], and an Incidence Density Ratio (IDR; game injury rate over practice injury rate) of 8.0 and 9.4, for boys and girls, respectively (p < 0.0001) [18]. Two additional high school studies provide further support by reporting the percentages of injuries in games and practices [19, 41]. Although no exposure data are provided, even a conservative estimate of 3 practices per game played indicate that the relative risk is approximately 2.2:1 for boys and between 2.1–2.8 for girls. Moreover, this relationship proved to be relatively consistent over time. Comparison of the 1986–1988 and 1995–1997 NATA [41] studies shows a game:practice relative risk for boys of 2.0 and 2.2, respectively, and 2.1 and 2.6 for girls, respectively (under the assumption of 3 practices per game played), although the risk in games may be rising for girls.

The higher risk of injuries in games is also reflected in data related to particular types of injuries in high school athletes, including orofacial injuries (1.8:1) [35] and MTBI IDR = 4.9 (95% CI: 2.9–8.1) for boys and 6.1 (95% CI: 3.8–9.7) for girls [33].

Two hospital-based studies, one from Denmark [48] and one from the USA [28], indicate that other situational factors need to be considered. Although both found that games and practices still accounted for the majority of basketball injuries seen (22.5 and 43%, respectively, in the Danish study and 42.9 and 37.5%, respectively, in the USA study), Sorensen et al. [48] found that free play or school activity accounted for 34.2% of the injuries treated, while Prebble et al. [28] noted that 9.6% came from physical education classes and 5.4% from intramurals or recess play.

Action or Activity

A broad set of actions has been identified in relation to injury in pediatric basketball, including colliding with another player (38.6%) [12]; (36.7%) [28]; (MTBI) [33], running (33%) [19, 25], shooting (29%) [19, 25], rebounding [19]; MTBI (girls) [33]; anterior cruciate ligament (ACL) injuries (88.55% boys; 60% girls) [49]; (26% boys; 30.8% girls) [41], twisting/turning (31.8%) [12], scrambling for loose balls (34.4% boys; 36.3% girls) [41] and controlled pattern activity (27.8% boys; 32.6% girls) [41].

A number of specific interactions have also been noted. Yde and Nielsen [25] found that, although only 29% of injuries occurred while shooting, it accounted for 60% of ankle injuries. Powell and Barber-Foss [19] found that boys had more shooting-related injuries in games whereas girls had more dribbling-related injuries. Piasecki et al. [49] reported that the majority of ACL injuries (62% for boys; 71% for girls) involved no contact with other players.

Chronometry

Few studies have documented the relationship of time factors to injuries. From the sparse information available, the risk of injury may be greater early in the season or late in games. A study of knee injuries in female high school programs found that most injuries occurred in the first half of the season [50]. The possible influence of fatigue as a risk factor is gleaned from studies in two disparate populations – 40.7% of all injuries in a YMCA program for young children occurred in last quarter of games [23], while a 3-year study of high school players found that 59% of injuries in boys' games and 63% in girls' games came in the second half [41].

Injury Severity

Injury Type

A percent comparison of injury types across high schools [17–19, 41], clubs/sporting organizations [23, 25–27], and hospital emergency departments [12, 29, 42, 43] is shown in table 3. Sprains [18, 19, 26, 27, 29, 41, 42] or sprains/strains [12, 17, 23, 28, 43] are the most common type of injury suffered by young basketball players, representing between 22–65.5% of all injuries. Strains account for approximately 16% of all reported injuries (range 13.3–17.7%) [19, 41]. Basketball players were more likely to sustain sprain or strains that any other sport monitored (football, baseball/softball, rollerblading/skating soccer, hockey) in a study at a large emergency department (OR = 2.6; 95% CI: 1.7–3.9) [12]. In a similar study, in a mixed sample (77.8% < age 19), 55.1% of basketball injuries were sprain/strains [28]. In a more in-depth analysis of knee injuries, de Loës et al. [30] found that in boys 21% of knee injuries were meniscal tears, 19% were ACL/posterior cruciate ligament (PCL) ruptures, 10% were medial/lateral collateral ligament tears and 32% were nonspecific ruptures. However, for girls, only 13% were meniscal tears with 18% ACL/PCL ruptures but 21% were medial/lateral collateral ligament tears. Patellar luxation was 13% of all knee injuries for girls compared to 4% for boys.

Overall, soft tissue injuries (contusions and abrasions) were the next most common type(s) of injuries reported, accounting for 15–36% of cases [17, 18, 23, 26, 29, 41, 43], although Belechri et al. [42] reported a range of 17.4–55% in five European countries. This group also reported the greatest percentage of fractures (17–36%), possibly due to the high number of hand/finger injuries reported. Generally, the range for fractures was 2.6–17.7% [17–19, 23, 26–28] although three studies reported fractures making up 26–28% of the total number of injuries [12, 29, 43]. Inflammatory conditions were rarely reported but Hickey et al. [27] found medial tibial stress syndrome to be responsible for 33.3% of all lower extremity injuries in a study of elite junior females, with patellar tendinopathy the most common knee problem (35.7%).

Table 3. A percent comparison of injury types in youth basketball players

Study	Number of participants	Number of injuries	Abrasions	Concussions/Neuro	Contusion	Luxations	Fractures	Inflammation	Lacerations	Nonspecific	Sprain	Strain	Other/Unknown
High schools													
Gomez et al. [17]	890 (girls)	436	–	2	15	2	6	–	2	–	56 (or strain)	–	14 (dental)
Messina et al. [18]	973 (boys)	543	–	2	20	3	5	–	9	–	47	–	14
	890 (girls)	436	–	2	15	2	6	–	2	–	56	–	17
Powell and Barber-Foss [19]	–	1,933 (boys)	–	2.8	–	–	8.6	–	–	26.6	44.8	15.1	2.2
	–	1,748 (girls)	–	3.6	–	–	6.8	–	–	22.8	45.1	17.7	4.0
NATA (1986–1988) [41]	? boys	?	–	–	22	–	–	–	–	–	43	–	65
	? girls	?	–	–	18	–	–	–	–	–	41	–	41
NATA (1995–1997) [41]	? boys	?	–	–	26.5	–	–	–	–	–	44.6	13.3	15.6
	? girls	?	–	–	19.6	–	–	–	–	–	44.2	16.2	20
Clubs/Sports organizations													
Gutgesell [23]	406 (boys)	39	–	–	35.9	–	2.6	–	5.1	–	28.2 (or strain)	–	28.2*
Yde and Nielsen [25]	56	21	–	–	–	–	–	–	–	–	–	–	–
de Loës [26]	15,095 (boys)	243	–	–	14.8	2.5	13.0	–	3.7	–	65.5	–	3.0
	10,154 (girls)	229	–	–	14.8	4.8	13.0	–	2.2	–	64.6	–	0.6
Hickey et al. [27]	49 (girls)	223[a]	–	–	–	–	9.3	10.3	–	6.3	21.9	–	3.6

Table 3 (continued)

Study	Number of participants	Number of injuries	Abrasions	Concussions/ Neuro	Contusion	Luxations	Fractures	Inflammation	Lacerations	Nonspecific	Sprain	Strain	Other/ Unknown
Emergency departments													
Taylor and Attia [12]	–	132	13.6% (or contusion)	–	–	–	28	–	5.3	–	48.5	– (or strain)	4.5
Damore et al. [29]	108 (patients)	111	1	–	19	5	28	–	–	1	47	–	–
Belechri et al. [42]													
(DEN)	?	257	33.9	0.8	(see abrasion)	38.9	19.5	–	1.9	5	(see luxations)	–	–
(FRA)	?	100	55	0.0	(see abrasion)	24	17	–	3	1	(see luxations)	–	–
(GRE)	?	856	49.5	1.2	(see abrasion)	21.7	20.9	–	4	2.7	(see luxations)	–	–
(NED)	?	2,000**	39	0.0	(see abrasion)	20	36	–	1	5	(see luxations)	–	–
(UK)	?	3,242**	17.4	0.5	(see abrasion)	20.3	20.7	–	5.3	35.8	(see luxations)	–	–
Finch et al. [43]	3,308	3,722	2.1	–	15.4	–	26.1	9.9	4.3	–	33.3 (or strain)	–	8.8

*Includes 12.8% epistaxis.
aPercentages for most common injuries only.
**Extrapolated to nationwide estimate.

Catastrophic Injury

Death or significant permanent disability is a powerful specter for parents and coaches of young basketball players. Fortunately, the risk of such events is small. Catastrophic injuries principally involve three body systems: central nervous system, cardiovascular system and respiratory system. In addition, significant permanent damage has been recorded for injuries to the eyes.

Although most brain and spine injuries occur from falling or colliding with fixed objects, other factors can be involved. For example, Tudor [51] describes a 17-year-old male player struck on the side of the head from a ball rebounding off the rim, producing an acute subdural hematoma with permanent disability including visual, emotional and behavioral deficits.

The most comprehensive picture of catastrophic injuries in pediatric basketball comes from the National Center for Catastrophic Sports Injuries (NCCSI) [52] which has been tracking these incidents in high school basketball programs in the USA since 1982. According to NCCSI, a catastrophic injury may be direct (brain/spinal cord injury or skull/spinal fracture) or indirect (systemic failure as a result of exertion in basketball or by a complication secondary to a non-fatal injury). In its 21st Annual report, NCCSI found that, in the period 1982–2003, there were 16 direct catastrophic injuries in this population, consisting of 2 fatalities (both male); 4 nonfatalities (permanent severe functional disability) and 10 serious injuries (no permanent disability but significant initial injuries, for example, vertebral fracture without paralysis). The direct injury fatality rate for males was 0.02 per 100,000 participants. For direct nonfatal injuries, the rate was 0.3 per 100,000 for males and 0.01 for females. For serious catastrophic injuries, the rate was 0.07 for males and 0.02 for females. However, there were 92 indirect catastrophic injuries during the same time producing 90 fatalities for a rate of 0.82 per 100,000 for males and 0.10 per 100,000 for females. Typically, indirect fatalities are cardiac failures [53]. No nonfatal injuries were recorded but the rate of indirect serious injuries was 0.01 per 100,000 for both males and females. The data in this report supercede several previous studies [53–55] but it is difficult to determine whether it captures all catastrophic injuries in high school-aged players. For example, those who may be injured in clubs.

Maron et al. [56] analyzed 134 cases of cardiovascular-related sudden deaths in trained athletes from 1985–1995: basketball accounted for 35%. The median age of fatalities was 17 (range 12–40), with 90% male. Hypertrophic cardiomyopathy was disproportionately prevalent in black athletes (48 vs. 26% of deaths; $p = 0.01$). Additional case reports indicate a variety of causal mechanisms. Serdaroglu et al. [57] commented on the case of a 15-year-old player who fell and developed multiple sensory and motor deficits. His condition deteriorated before a rupture of the descending aorta was diagnosed and treated surgically but without success. Messina et al. [18] implicated pulmonary 'complications' subsequent to a thigh contusion in the death of a 16-year-old male player.

The most important respiratory complication appears to be related to asthma. A recent 7-year study of asthma-related fatalities in sport [58] found that of 61 deaths most occurred in athletes aged under 20 (prevalent group 10–14), with basketball one of the two most frequent activities precipitating a fatal episode (track was the other).

Finally, a series of case reports indicate that significant and permanent damage to the eyes can arise from fingers or the ball penetrating the orbit. Of particular concern are avulsions of the optic nerve, at least 7 cases of which are reported in the literature [59, 60].

Time Loss

If advances in playing safety are to occur, understanding the circumstances of injuries that result in time away from playing or normal life activities, such as school, is critical. A summary of time-loss studies is shown in table 4 [15, 20, 23, 25, 28, 31, 33, 41, 48, 61–63]. Unfortunately, the variety of data sources (clubs, schools, hospitals), player attributes (gender, age) and sociocultural characteristics (nationality, urban) make it difficult to get a clear picture of the risk of significant (i.e., time loss) injuries in pediatric basketball. Moreover, actual time-loss data are provided in only a limited number of studies although some information on time loss can be extrapolated from injury-severity data.

For example, Gutgesell [23] noted that only 2.4% of injuries in a YMCA program with children aged 5–12 resulted in missed playing time but did not provide any further details. In a study in a Danish sports club involving players up to the age of 18, 43% of time-loss injuries were resolved in less than 2 weeks with a further 33% resolved by 4 weeks. No case took longer than 6 weeks to resolve [25].

In an early high school study, McLain and Reynolds [15] found that the mean time lost for a basketball injury for boys was 11.8 days but 28.6 days for girls. However, the authors noted that there were only 45 girls in the study, and one sustained an ACL rupture necessitating surgical reconstruction and was absent for almost a full year. Removing this case from the data brought the girls' average time-loss due to injury to 7.8 days. The influence of a single significant injury on outcomes such as the mean days lost when the pool is small is problematic. Similarly, Axe et al. [61] undertook a 1-year prospective study of adolescent sports injuries reporting to a Delaware sports clinic: female basketball players averaged 12.8 days lost per injury (28 cases with 3 surgeries) compared to 9.2 days for boys (20 cases with one surgery). As above, one female case was a season-ending ACL rupture (110 days lost) and removing this from the tally reduced average days lost for girls to 8.8.

Table 4. Summary of injury-related time loss in youth basketball

Study	Number of injuries	Age	Situation	Time loss
McLain and Reynolds [15]	21 (boys) 14 (girls)	15–18	High school	Boys: 11.8 days (mean); Girls: 28.6 days (mean) (w/o 1 ACL case, girls' mean: 7.8 days)
Beachey et al. [20]	505 (boys) 467 (girls)	Grades 7–12	High school	Boys: 31% > 1 day Girls: 37% > 1 day
Gutgesell [23]	39 (boys/girls)	5–12	YMCA	2.4% missed playing time
Yde and Nielsen [25]	21 (boys/girls)	<18	Club	43% < 2 weeks; 33% 2–4 weeks; 24% 4–6 weeks
Prebble et al. [28]	1,210	77.8% 10–19	ED (USA)	71.2% < 14 days
McGuine et al. [31] (ankle only)	23 (boys/girls)	15–18	High school	56.5% < 7 days; 39.1% 7–21 days; 4.3% > 21 days; 7.1 days (mean)
Powell and Barber-Foss [33] (MTBI only)	1,219	15–18	High school	Boys: 88.2% < 8 days; 9.8% 8–21 days; 2.0% > 21 days Girls: 83.1% < 8 days; 13.8% 8–21 days; 3.1% > 21 days
NATA [41]	?	15–18	High school	Boys: 79.4% < 7 days; 12.4% 7–21 days; 8.2% > 21 days Girls: 76% < 7 days; 15% 7–21 days; 9.0% > 21 days
Sorenson et al. [48]	57 (boys) 54 (girls)	6–17 6–17	ED (DEN)	Boys: mean 5.4 days (range 0–45 days) from training Boys: mean 1.5 days (range 0–20 days) from school Girls: mean 4.2 days (range 0–40 days) from training Girls: mean 0.3 days (range 0–5 days) from school
Axe et al. [61]	20 (boys) 28 (girls)	14–18	Clinic	Boys: 9.2 days (mean); Girls: 12.8 days (mean) (w/o 1 ACL case, girls' mean: 8.8 days)
Rider and Hicks [62]	52 (boys/girls)	15–18	High school	96% < 7 days; mean = 3.1 days
Watson [63]	9	10–18	Elementary/HS	BB > than mean for all sports for hospitalization (0.47 days; 18 days out)

Data from several other high school studies provide a mixed picture. Rider and Hicks [62] found that, in a study of male and female high school varsity players over one season, 27% missed at least one day due to injury but only 4% missed more than 7 days. The average for the group was 3.1 days. Beachey et al. [20] noted that, over an 8-year period, 31% of injuries to boys in a single high school team resulted in at least one day lost from practice, while about 37% of injuries to girls were time-loss, although no information on average time-loss or the range was provided. In a 3-year study involving a national sample of high schools, the National Athletic Trainers Association (NATA) [41] found that 79.4% of boys' injuries and 76% of girls' injuries could be considered minor (<7 days absent) with only 8.2% for boys and 9.0% for girls being major (requiring more than 21 days).

However, in a one-year study of Irish school children aged 10–18, Watson [63] found that, while basketball accounted for only 7.7% of the injuries recorded (9 of 116), these 'tended to result in an above average period of hospitalization and incapacity' (average period of hospitalization for all sports was 0.47 days with 18 days of incapacity). The author suggests that the difference with American data may be sociocultural in that 'Irish teachers and coaches are reluctant to classify an incident as an 'injury' unless the level of incapacity is high and they tend to ignore conditions that would be referred for medical treatment in America, where the level of involvement of medical and paramedical personnel in sport is considerably greater' (p 70).

School-based studies of the severity of particular types of injuries have also been published. Powell and Barber-Foss [33] examined MTBI in male and female athletes in 235 USA high schools and found that 5.5% of all reported injuries in 10 sports over 3 years were MTBI with boys and girls basketball accounting for 4.2% (51 cases) and 5.2% (63 cases) of the total, respectively. Most cases were minor (resolved in <8 days) in 88.2 and 83.1% of cases for boys and girls, respectively, with only 2 and 3.1%, respectively, taking more than 21 days. In a prospective study investigating balance characteristics on the risk of ankle injury, McGuine et al. [31] found that 56.5% of reported ankle injuries in the study group of 210 male and female athletes resolved in less than 7 days while 39.1% took 7–21 days. Only one injury (4.3%) took longer than 21 days to resolve.

Finally, information from several hospital-based studies, which theoretically should involve more severe cases, indicates that the bulk of basketball injuries are minor. Finch et al. [43] found that, although basketball was the fourth leading cause of sports-related injuries in a 4-year national study of emergency departments, it ranked ninth (of ten) in subsequent hospital admissions. In a study in rural America, Prebble et al. [28] found that 71.2% of cases seen at an emergency department resolved in less than 2 weeks. In contrast, a more extensive study from Denmark [48] found that basketball injuries resulted in an average time away from training of 5.4 days (range 0–45 days) for boys and 4.2 days (range 0–40) for girls. However, the time absent from school was only 1.5 days (range 0–20) for boys and 0.3 days (range 0–5 days) for girls, indicating that the limitations were activity-specific rather than generally debilitating.

Clinical Outcome

In line with the limited amount of quality data on more direct issues related to understanding the nature and risk of basketball injuries, very little research has been performed on the associated costs of injuries, such as the financial impact (both direct and indirect) on individuals, sponsoring organizations, and national associations. Although improvements in playing safety can arise from altruistic concerns, progress tends to come from the impact of pragmatic issues such as the influence of injuries on insurance costs, days lost from work or school, or the drain on medical resources. For example, in a 7-year study of only knee injuries in a national sample of 14–20-year-old male and female players in Switzerland, de Loës et al. [30] found that the mean medical cost for treatment of knee injuries (including ACL/PCL ruptures) was USD 1,427 for males and USD 1,060 for females. These costs were in the context of a national insurance program. By contrast, Hewett et al. [64] estimated that the cost of reconstruction and rehabilitation of an ACL rupture in a female high school basketball player in the USA is at least USD 17,000, producing a total direct financial impact of more than USD 119 million per year for this population alone [65]. If only 1% of the costs were available for research on injury analysis and prevention, substantial advances could be made in reducing the human, financial, and medical burden of basketball injuries in youth and adolescent players. Similarly, Newsome et al. [66] reported that the lifetime dental costs of a tooth avulsion that is not properly preserved or replanted can be more than USD 10,000 but custom-fitted mouthguards that can reduce the risk significantly can be made available for less than USD 10 [67].

Injury Risk Factors

Intrinsic Factors

Gender

Despite the widely varying quality of the literature dealing with injuries in youth basketball, girls are more at risk than boys, particularly for knee and ankle injuries, and these injuries tend to be serious [14, 16, 18, 19, 23, 26, 30, 32, 41, 49, 68]. This relationship has been noted in club [23, 26, 30] and scholastic studies [14, 16, 32, 41, 49, 68], in the USA [14, 16, 18, 32, 41, 49, 68] and abroad [26, 30]. Several studies have found no overall gender difference in injury data [18, 19, 25] but still noted significant differences in the number of knee injuries between boys and girls [18, 19].

Specifically, although several high school studies did not find a significant difference in overall injury rates between boys and girls ($p = 0.11$) [18], IDR $= 1.01, 95\%$ CI $= 0.95–1.08$ [19], there is a gender-related risk ($p < 0.05$) [26], ($p < 0.02$) [23], ($p < 0.001$) [14], ($p < 0.0004$) [16]. In addition, although Gutgesell [23] found a similar rate of serious injury between boys and girls, others identified a significant difference in this outcome ($p < 0.05$) [19]; ($p < 0.001$) [14], with Chandy and Grana [14] noting a significantly greater number of season-ending injuries for girls ($p < 0.001$).

Of the available literature, girls are at a greater risk of sustaining a knee injury ($p < 0.001$) [14]; (IDR $= 1.44; 95\%$ CI: $1.2–1.71$) [19]; (IDR 1.7, $p < 0.05$) [30]; (RR $1.92, p < 0.0001$) [32]; (RR $2.29, p < 0.001$) [18], and the knee injury is more likely to require surgery ($p < 0.05$) [14]; (IDR $= 2.65, 95\%$ CI $= 1.64–4.29$) [19]; ($p < 0.047$) [18] and/or involve the ACL (RR $= 9.0$, $p = 0.05$) [49]; (RR $= 3.79, p < 0.024$) [18]; ($p < 0.01$) [68]; (IDR $= 4.14$, 95% CI: $2.18–7.9$) [19]. However, Piasecki et al. [49] noted that girls seem to be at less risk for medial femoral condyle injuries ($p = 0.05$).

Girls also seem to be at greater risk than boys of sustaining an ankle injury (RR $= 1.24, p < 0.05$) [32] and being reinjured ($p = 0.002$) [19].

Age and Development

There is conflicting information about the influence of age and/or level of development on injury in young players. Yde and Nielsen [25] concluded that the risk of injury increases with age, while DuRant et al. [16] did not. However, Michaud et al. [11] reported that the risk appears to increase with pubertal development (Tanner stage 4 or 5) rather than chronological age. A study of five European Union nations [42] showed a consistent increase in the percentage of basketball injuries with age. Although this may be simply a reflection of increasing participation rates, it probably also captures the influence of physical development on injuries as players become larger, stronger and faster. The percentage of all basketball injuries represented by 5–8 year olds ranged from 1% in France to 5.4% in the United Kingdom; for those 9–10 from 4% in France to 16% in Greece; 11–12 from 23% in France to 39.3% in Denmark; and for 13–14 year olds from 42.9% in Greece to 72% in France.

Psychological Characteristics

Despite the importance of psychological factors on performance, few studies have examined the relationship between mental states and injury. Only two studies dealt with these issues in young basketball players. In a study conducted in the late 1970s with female high school players, Young and Cohen [69] found that injured players were significantly different from uninjured players on several psychological measures, including total self-concept, self-criticism, and in measures of external frames of reference, indicating they may be inherently 'risk-takers'. In a more recent study no relationship was found between psychological factors related to life-stress events, coping skills and social support and time-loss due to injury [62].

Other Factors

As the effort to reduce injury rates in youth basketball continues, researchers have focused on a diverse range of potential risk factors, including proprioceptive ability [31], level of motor development [39], level of competition [32], and influence of fixed orthodontic appliances [35].

McGuine et al. [31] examined the relationship between a standardized balance test and ankle injury, and found a positive linear relationship between postural sway (measured in degrees per second) and rate of ankle injuries per 1,000 AE. Kelm et al. [39] reported that more than 50% of all basketball injuries in physical education classes involving 11–15 year olds involved catching, implicating poor motor skills, including hand/eye coordination, as a risk factor.

In a 2-year prospective study with matched boys and girls high school and college programs, Hosea et al. [32] found that the relative risk of injury increased with level of competition (from high school to college), doubling for both boys and girls. However, for ACL injuries specifically, the relative risk was significant for girls (3.66:1; p < 0.01) but not boys moving to collegiate competition.

Finally, Kvettem et al. [35] noted a relative risk of orofacial injury while wearing a fixed orthodontic appliance of 1.7 (95% CI = 1.1–2.5), although the small sample warrants caution in interpreting the data.

Extrinsic Factors

Few studies have attempted to identify play-related factors that impact injury potential. Data from two studies [33, 50] indicate that playing guard is more hazardous than playing forward. In a report of knee injuries in 22 female high school basketball programs in Iowa, guards had 3 times as many knee ligament tears as forwards [50]. In addition, guards were most at risk for game-related MTBI (62.5% boys; 56.4% girls), although forwards accounted for most MTBI injuries in practice (68.4% boys; 62.5% girls) [33].

Addressing a common situation in community-based programs, Gutgesell [23] found that for young children playing on a linoleum-tile playing surface was not more hazardous than playing on a standard wood floor.

Suggestions for Injury Prevention

Despite the dearth of definitive information on risk factors related to youth basketball, a variety of recommendations have been presented based on the limited research and general observations and which take into account the unique characteristics of young players. A summary of the recommendations indicating the study design of the resources from which the recommendations were drawn is shown in table 5 [14, 16, 19, 22, 25, 31, 34–36, 39, 40, 46, 59, 60, 63–67, 70–73]. The majority are 'common sense' responses to apparent cause-effect relationships and cover multiple aspects of playing basketball. Although few have been empirically tested, the general principle on which they are based, i.e., modifying the rigors of the game and/or the physical capacities of the players to better match, is not unreasonable and has some research support. A summary of prevention studies is shown in table 6 [31, 62, 64, 69, 71, 72, 74–76].

Injury prevention studies are predictive or remedial. On the premise that it is better to prevent than correct an injury, identifying predictive characteristics should be a primary research goal. Studies, covering physical (balance, structural symmetry, tenderness) and psychological (self-concept, coping skills) factors, have had mixed success. However, because of methodological problems, including limited sample sizes, it is unclear whether factors that found to have no predictive value in fact are not related to injury, or whether the relationship is masked by design flaws. In some cases, implementation of predictive or screening protocols is hampered by logistical issues such as cost and the need for specialized equipment. Hewett et al.'s [64] remedial intervention program of neuromuscular training to reduce the incidence of knee injuries is the most promising as it is designed to complement normal basketball conditioning programs.

Suggestions for Further Research

The lack of clear comprehensive data on injuries in youth basketball is distressing considering that it is one of the most popular sports in the world and the number of young participants is rising, as is the personal, financial and social burden of basketball injuries. The options for future research are numerous, and fall into three broad categories: (1) development of appropriate research programs in general, (2) research into specific risk factors, and (3) research into the characteristics of specific injuries.

If any significant progress is to be made in understanding the determinants of injury in this population, a fundamental retooling of the structure of the

Table 5. Suggestions for injury prevention

Preventive measure	Reference	Type of evidence
Environmental issues		
Develop basic motor skills in new/young players	Yde and Nielsen [25]	Prospective cohort
	Watson [63]	Prospective cohort
Modify playing conditions to players' skill level	Yde and Nielsen [25]	Prospective cohort
(court and ball size, number of players, etc)	Kelm et al. [39]	Case series
Reduce size of physical education classes for better instruction/supervision	Backx et al. [22]	Prospective cohort
Ensure well-trained officials	DuRant et al. [16]	Prospective cohort
	Watson [63]	Prospective cohort
Ensure players matched in physical characteristics/skill	DuRant et al. [16]	Prospective cohort
Protective equipment and conditions		
Educate parents, coaches, players about mouth guard use*	Maestrello-deMoya and Primosch [34]	Retrospective cohort
	Kvettem et al. [35]	Prospective cohort
	Teo et al. [36]	Retrospective cohort
	Diab and Mourino [46]	Cross-sectional
	Newsome et al. [66]	Review
	McNutt et al. [70]	Cross-sectional
	Foster and March [71]	Quasi-experimental field study
	Jalleh [72]	Quasi-experimental field study
Develop methods to supply inexpensive custom mouthguard**	Johnson and Parker [67]	Implementation project
Campaign for mandatory mouthguard use	Foster and March [71]	Quasi-experimental field study
Encourage voluntary mouthguard use	Teo et al. [36]	Retrospective cohort
Encourage use of protective eyewear	Chow et al. [59]	Case study
	Friedman [60]	Case study

Table 5 (continued)

Preventive measure	Reference	Type of evidence
Ensure coaches have first aid training	Backx et al. [40]	Prospective cohort
Ensure that high schools have NATA-certified athletic trainers	AAFP [73]	Policy statement
Engage injured athletes in well constructed rehabilitation programs	McGuine et al. [31]	Prospective cohort
Player attributes		
Implement developmentally appropriate preparticipation fitness evaluations	Chandy and Grana [14]	Retrospective cohort
Implement developmentally appropriate conditioning programs (strength, agility, flexibility, power)	Chandy and Grana [14]	Retrospective cohort
	DuRant et al. [16]	Prospective cohort
	Backx et al. [22]	Prospective cohort
	Watson [63]	Prospective cohort
Instigate specific ankle stabilization/proprioception training	Powell and Barber-Foss [19]	Retrospective cohort
	Backx et al. [22]	Prospective cohort
Instigate specific ACL dynamic neuromuscular training***	Hewett et al. [64]	Prospective cohort
(especially for girls)	Ford et al. [65]	Laboratory study

*A complete team and community educational program is available from Sports Medicine Australia (Western Australia Branch). This program has been demonstrated to be effective in significantly increasing mouthguard use in young basketball players. For further details refer to Foster and March [71] and Jalleh et al. [72].

**Refer to Johnson and Parker [67] for a description of a project that supplied custom-fitted mouthguards to three high school teams for under $10 each.

***Refer to Hewett et al. [64] for a description of a program shown to significantly reduce the incidence of serious knee injuries.

Harmer

Table 6. Summary of injury prevention studies

Reference	Design	Participants	Intervention	Outcome variable	Results
McGuine et al. [31]	Prospective cohort	High school (n = 210)	Postural sway measures	Ankle injuries	Athletes with high sway scores 7 times risk of ankle injury (p = 0.0002)
Rider and Hicks [62]	Prospective cohort	High school (n = 67)	Psychological measures of life events stress, coping skills, social support	Injury	No predictive value in these measures
Hewett et al. [64]	Nonrandomized clinical trial	High school (n = 498)	Jump training, stretching, weight training	Serious knee injuries	Trained: fewer noncontact knee injuries (p = 0.019)
Young and Cohen [69]	Prospective cohort	High school (n = 190)	Psychological measures of self-concept	Injury	Total self-concept, self-criticism, identity, personal self & physical scale scores significantly different between injured and non-injured players (p < 0.1)
Foster and March [71] Jalleh et al. [72]	Quasi-experimental field study	Club (pre: n = 1,429) (post: n = 1,148)	Mouthguard education program	Mouthguard use	Use increased significantly – Competition: OR = 2.55 (95% CI: 2.04–3.18) Training: OR = 4.39 (95% CI: 3.21–6.00)
Grubbs et al. [74]	Nonrandomized clinical trial	High school (n = 62)	Structural symmetry measures	Lower extremity injuries	No predictive value in these measures
Cook et al. [75]	Prospective cohort	Club (n = 26)	Ultrasonography of patellar tendon	Patellar symptoms	Ultrasonographic hypoechoic area associated with patellar tendinitis (p < 0.05) but baseline values not predictive of outcome
Cook et al. [76]	Correlational	Club (n = 163)	Palpation of patellar tendon	Patellar tendinitis	Patellar tenderness is not a useful in preparticipation examinations as screening method

research, utilizing appropriate epidemiological methods, is necessary. A number of authors have commented on such basic considerations as the need to establish standards for an unambiguous definition of reportable injury and denominator data (exposure information), and the use of trained professionals, such as certified athletic trainers with standardized recording systems, to develop the data for analysis [19, 25, 26], within a coordinated series of regional and national databases [68].

Identifying risk and protective factors associated with the diverse characteristics of the pediatric population remains a high priority. Issues such as age, level of competition, developmental status, and the influence of various types of training programs or psychological and social factors on injury characteristics remain to be explored [18, 62], as does the need to establish standardized protocols for measuring intrinsic characteristics, such as postural sway, as predictors of injury [31].

Of the specific types of injuries that can occur in basketball, clearly research to reduce the incidence of knee and ankle injuries must be a high priority [27]. This is of particular importance for young female participants in light of the consistent indications of their vulnerability to these injuries. Additionally, several authors have indicated the need to continue research on orofacial injuries and mouthguard protection [34, 35], which has already yielded important advances in significantly reducing these problems.

Finally, there is a need to acknowledge basketball as a global phenomenon and that the determinants of safe play may be moderated by cultural considerations. Regional interests must be addressed in the study of short- and long-term consequences of basketball injuries in young athletes [9].

References

1   Fédération Internationale de Basketball (FIBA): Quick facts. 2004;www.fiba.com
2   National Federation of State High School Associations (NFHS): Participation sets record for sixth straight year. Press release Aug 24, 2004;www.nfhs.org
3   MMWR: Nonfatal sports- and recreation-related injuries treated in emergency departments – United States, July 2000 – June 2001. MMWR 2002;51:736–740.
4   American Academy of Orthopaedic Surgeons: A guide to safety for young athletes 2002; www.orthoinfo.aaos.org/brochure.
5   National SAFE KIDS Campaign (NSKC): Sports injury fact sheet 2004. Washington DC, NSKC, 2004.
6   Zvijac J, Thompson W: Basketball; in Caine DJ, Caine CG, Lindner KJ (eds): Epidemiology of Sports Injuries. Champaign, Human Kinetics, 1996.
7   Watkins J, Peabody P: Sports injuries in children and adolescents at a sports injury clinic. J Sports Med Phys Fitness 1996;36:43–48.
8   Boyce SH, Quigley MA: An audit of sports injuries in children attending an Accident & Emergency department. Scott Med J 2003;48:88–90.

9 Maffulli N, Bundoc RC, Chan KM, Cheng JCY: Paediatric sports injuries in Hong Kong: A seven year survey. Br J Sports Med 1996;30:218–221.

10 Frontera WR, Micheo WF, Amy E, Melédez E, Aguirre G, Correa JJ, Camunas JF: Patterns of injury in athletes evaluated in an interdisciplinary clinic. PR Health Sci J 1994;13:165–170.

11 Michaud P-A, Renaud A, Narring F: Sports activities related to injuries? A survey among 9–19 year olds in Switzerland. Inj Prev 2001;7:41–45.

12 Taylor B, Attia MW: Sports-related injuries in children. Acad Emerg Med 2000;7:1366–1382.

13 Gordis L: Epidemiology. Philadelphia, Saunders, 2000.

14 Chandy TA, Grana WA: Secondary school athletic injuries in boys and girls: A three-year comparison. Phys Sportsmed 1985;13:106–111.

15 McLain LG, Reynolds S: Sports injuries in a high school. Pediatrics 1989;84:446–450.

16 DuRant RH, Pendergrast RA, Seymore C, Gaillard G, Donner J: Findings from the Preparticipation Athletic Examination and athletic injuries. Am J Dis Child 1992;146:85–91.

17 Gomez E, DeLee JC, Farney WC: Incidence of injury in Texas girls' high school basketball. Am J Sports Med 1996;24:684–687.

18 Messina DF, Farney WC, DeLee JC: The incidence of injury in Texas high school basketball. A prospective study among male and female athletes. Am J Sports Med 1999;27:294–299.

19 Powell JW, Barber-Foss KD: Sex-related injury patterns among selected high school sports. Am J Sports Med 2000;28:385–391.

20 Beachy G, Akau CK, Martinson M, Olderr TF: A longitudinal study at Punahou School: 1988 to 1996. Am J Sports Med 1997;25:675–681.

21 Weir MA, Watson AWS: A twelve month study of sports injuries in one Irish school. Ir J Med Sci 1996;165:165–169.

22 Backx FJ, Beijer HJ, Bol E, Erich WB: Injuries in high-risk persons and high-risk sports – A longitudinal study of 18118 school children. Am J Sports Med 1991;19:124–130.

23 Gutgesell ME: Safety of a preadolescent basketball program. Am J Dis Child 1991;145:1023–1025.

24 Chambers RB: Orthopaedic injuries in athletes (ages 6 to 17). Am J Sports Med 1979;7:195–197.

25 Yde J, Nielsen AB: Sports injuries in adolescents' ball games: Soccer, handball and basketball. Br J Sports Med 1990;24:51–54.

26 de Loës M: Epidemiology of sports injuries in the Swiss Organization 'Youth and Sports' 1987–1989. Int J Sports Med 1995;16:134–138.

27 Hickey GJ, Fricker PA, McDonald WA: Injuries to young elite basketball players over a six-year period. Clin J Sport Med 1997;7:252–256.

28 Prebble T, Chyou P-H, Wittman L, McCormick J, Collins K, Zoch T: Basketball injuries in a rural area. Wis Med J 1999;98:22–24.

29 Damore DT, Metzl JD, Ramundo M, Pan S, van Amerongen, R: Patterns in childhood sports injury. Pediatr Emerg Care 2003;19:65–67.

30 de Loes M, Dahlstedt LJ, Thomee R: A 7-year study on risks and costs of knee injuries in male and female youth participants in 12 sports. Scand J Med Sci Sports 2000;10:90–97.

31 McGuine TA, Greene JJ, Best T, Leverson G: Balance as a predictor of ankle injuries in high school basketball players. Clin J Sport Med 2000;10:239–244

32 Hosea TM, Carey CC, Harrer MF: The gender issue: Epidemiology of ankle injuries in athletes who participate in basketball. Clin Ortho Rel Res 2000;372:45–49.

33 Powell JW, Barber-Foss KD: Traumatic brain injury in high school athletes. JAMA 1999;282:958–963.

34 Maestrello-deMoya MG, Primosch RE: Orofacial trauma and mouth-protector wear among high school varsity basketball players. J Dent Child 1989;1:36–39.

35 Kvittem B, Hardie NA, Roettger M, Conry J: Incidence of orofacial injuries in high school sport. J Public Health Dent 1998;58:288–293.

36 Teo CS, Stokes AN, Loh T, Bagramin RA: A survey of tooth injury experience and attitudes to prevention in a group of Singapore schoolboys. Ann Acad Med 1995;24:23–25.

37 Burt CW, Overpeck MD: Emergency visits for sports-related injuries. Ann Emerg Med 2001;37:301–308.

38 Conn JM, Annest JL, Gilchrist J: Sports and recreation related injury episodes in the US population, 1997–99. Inj Prev 2003;9:117–123.

39   Kelm J, Ahelm F, Pape D, Pitsch W, Engel C: School sports accidents: Analysis of causes, modes, and frequencies. J Pediatr Orthop 2001;21:165–168.
40   Backx FJ, Erich WB, Kemper AB, Verbeek AL: Sports injuries in school-aged children – An epidemiological study. Am J Sports Med 1989;17:234–240.
41   National Athletic Trainers Association (NATA): 1995–1997 injury surveillance overview. NATA 2004;www.nata.org/publications/otherpubs/injuryinformaiton.htm
42   Belechri M, Petridou E, Kedikolglou S, Trichopoulos D, 'Sports Injuries' European Union Group: Sports injuries among children in six European Union countries. Eur J Epidemiol 2001;17: 1005–1012.
43   Finch C, Valuri G, Ozanne-Smith J: Sport and active recreation injuries in Australia: Evidence from emergency department presentations. Br J Sports Med 1998;32:220–225.
44   Macgregor DM: Don't save the ball. Br J Sports Med 2003;37:351–353.
45   Sane J: Comparison of maxillofacial and dental injuries in four contact team sports: American football, bandy, basketball, and handball. Am J Sports Med 1988;16:647–652.
46   Diab N, Mourino AP: Parental attitudes towards mouthguards. Pediatr Dent 1997;19:455–460.
47   Wan J, Corvino TF, Greenfield SP, DiScala C: Kidney and testicle injuries in team and individual sports: Data from the National Pediatric Trauma Registry. J Urol 2003;170:1528–1532.
48   Sorenson L, Larsen SE, Rock ND: Sports injuries in school-aged children – A study of traumatological and socioeconomic outcome. Scand J Med Sci Sports 1998;8:52–56.
49   Piasecki DP, Spindler KP, Warren TA, Andrish JT, Parker RD: Intraarticular injuries associated with anterior cruciate ligament tear: Findings at ligament reconstruction in high school and recreational athletes. Am J Sports Med 2003;31:601–605.
50   Wirtz PD: High school basketball knee ligament injuries. J Iowa med Soc 1982;72:105–106.
51   Tudor RB: Acute subdural hematoma following a blow from a basketball. Am J Sports Med 1979;7:136.
52   National Center for Catastrophic Sport Injury (NCCSI): 21st Annual report. NCCSI 2004; www.unc.edu/depts/nnccsi/ReportDataTables.htm.
53   Mueller FO, Cantu RC: Catastrophic injuries and fatalities in high school and college sports, fall 1982-spring 1988. Med Sci Sports Exerc 1990;22:737–741.
54   Mueller FO: Catastrophic head injuries in high school and collegiate sports. J Athl Train 2001;36:312–315.
55   Maron BJ, Gohman TE, Aeppli D: Prevalence of sudden cardiac death during competitive sports activities in Minnesota high school athletes. J Am Coll Cardiol 1998;32:1881–1884.
56   Maron BJ, Shirani J, Poliac LC, Mathenge R, Roberts WC, Meuller FO: Sudden death in young competitive athletes: Clinical, demographic and pathological profiles. JAMA 1996;276:199–204.
57   Serdaroglu G, Levent E, Yurtseve S, Calkavur T, Yunten N, Aydogdu S: Dissection of aorta: A pediatric case report. Turk J Pediatr 2002;44:254–257.
58   Becker JM, Rogers J, Rossini G, Mirchandani H, D'Alonzo GE: Asthma deaths during sports: Report of a 7-year experience. J Allergy Clin Immunol 2004;113:264–267.
59   Chow AY, Goldberg MF, Frenkel M: Evulsion of the optic nerve in association with basketball injuries. Ann Ophthalmol 1984;16:35–37.
60   Friedman SM: Optic nerve avulsion secondary to a basketball injury. Ophthalmic Surg Lasers 1999;30:676–677.
61   Axe MJ, Newcomb WA, Warner D: Sports injuries and adolescent athletes. Del Med J 1991;63: 359–363.
62   Rider SP, Hicks RA: Stress, coping and injuries in male and female high school basketball players. Percept Mot Skills 1995;81:499–503.
63   Watson AWS: Sports injuries during one academic year in 6799 Irish school children. Am J Sports Med 1984;12:65–71.
64   Hewett TE, Riccobene JV, Lindenfeld TN, Noyes FR: The effect of neuromuscular training on the incidence of knee injury in female athletes: A prospective study. Am J Sports Med 1999;27:699–706.
65   Ford KR, Myer GD, Hewett TE: Valgus knee motion during landing in high school female and male basketball players. Med Sci Sports Exerc 1999;35:1745–1750.
66   Newsome PRH, Tran DC, Cooke MS: The role of the mouthguard in the prevention of sports-related dental injuries: A review. Int J Paediatr Dent 2001;11:396–404.

67   Johnson DW, Parker BJ: Athletic mouth guards – One town's approach. J Calif Dent Assoc 1993;21:39–42.
68   Micheli LJ, Metzl JD, DiCanzio J, Zurakowski D: Anterior cruciate ligament reconstructive surgery in adolescent soccer and basketball players. Clin J Sport Med 1999;9:138–141.
69   Young ML, Cohen DA: Self-concept and injuries among high school basketball players. J Sports Med 1981;21:55–61.
70   McNutt T, Shannon SW, Wright JT, Feinstein RA: Oral trauma in adolescent athletes: A study of mouth protectors. Pediatr Dent 1989;11:209–213.
71   Foster M, March K: Increasing mouthguard use. A pilot campaign for junior basketball and rugby. Aust Endod J 1999;25:87–89.
72   Jalleh G, Donovan RJ, Clarkson J, March K, Foster M, Giles-Corti B: Increasing mouthguard usage among junior rugby and basketball players. Aus NZJ Public Health 2001;25:250–252.
73   American Academy of Family Physicians: Policy statement – Sports medicine 2004;www.aafp.org.
74   Grubbs N, Nelson RT, Bandy WD: Predictive validity of an injury score among high school basketball players. Med Sci Sports Exerc 1997;29:1279–1285.
75   Cook JL, Khan KM, Kiss ZS, Purdam CR, Griffiths L: Prospective imaging study of asymptomatic patellar tendinopathy in elite junior basketball players. J Ultrasound Med 2000;19:473–479.
76   Cook JL, Khan KM, Kiss ZS, Purdam CR, Griffiths L: Reproducibility and clinical utility of tendon palpation to detect patellar tendinopathy in young basketball players. Br J Sports Med 2001;35:65–69.

Professor Peter Harmer
Exercise Science-Sports Medicine
Willamette University, Salem, OR 97301 (USA)
Tel. +1 503 370 6470, Fax +1 503 370 6379, E-Mail pharmer@willamette.edu

Maffulli N, Caine DJ (eds): Epidemiology of Pediatric Sports Injuries: Team Sports.
Med Sport Sci. Basel, Karger, 2005, vol 49, pp 62–85

....

Gridiron Football Injuries

Michael J. Stuart

The Mayo Clinic, Department of Orthopedic Surgery, Rochester, Minn., USA

Abstract

Objective: To review the available football epidemiology literature to identify risk factors, facilitate injury prevention and uncover deficiencies that may be addressed by future research. **Data Sources:** A literature search of Sports Discus (1940–2003), Eric (1967–2003), EMBASE (1988–2003), MEDLINE (1966–2003), CINAHL (1984–2003), and Web of Science (1993–2003) identified the published articles on American football in athletes of high school age and younger. **Main Results:** Injury rate increases with the level of play (grade in school), player age, and player experience. The lower extremity (knee and ankle joints) is most frequently injured. Football injuries are much more common in games than in practice, and occur to players who are being tackled, tackling or blocking. Most injuries are mild, including contusion, strain and sprain. Rule changes with the prohibition of initial contact with the helmet or face-mask reduced catastrophic head and neck injuries. **Conclusion:** Although no sport or recreational activity is completely risk-free, football epidemiology research is critical to injury prevention. The existing medical literature provides some valuable insights, but an increased emphasis on prospective research is required to test the efficacy of preventative measures. Quality research may contribute to a reduction in football injury risk by defining the role of player conditioning and strength training, coaching of safety fundamentals, avoidance of dangerous activities, as well as proper medical supervision and care. Sports medicine personnel, coaches, and officials must strive to minimize injuries through progressive education, improved coaching techniques, effective officiating, and equipment modifications.

Introduction

Thirty-five million children and young adults in the United States participate in sports [1]. One of every fourteen teenagers presenting to the emergency room following a traumatic event has a sports-related injury, and American football is the most common precipitating athletic activity [2]. Approximately 1.2 million injuries occur each year as a result of 1.5 million athletes participating in organized American football [3]. The knee and ankle are most commonly injured in this collision and contact team sport, but football has also been associated with catastrophic injuries involving the brain and cervical spine [4].

The sports medicine community has attempted to document the risks and the mechanisms of injury in the game of gridiron football, especially concussion, spinal cord trauma and death [3, 5–11]. The nature of available reports range from surveys, which estimate the absolute number of injuries, to prospective cohort analyses that identify risk factors and suggest preventative measures [12–15]. The bulk of the literature concerning gridiron football injuries has focused on the high school age athlete and older [8, 11, 15–22]. Few studies have investigated the risk of participation in American football at the youth level, but injury rate and severity appears surprisingly low when compared to those competitors who have passed through puberty [14, 21, 23–27].

Problem Statement

A review of American football epidemiology research permits administrators, sports medicine professionals, coaches and players to identify risk factors and hopefully facilitate injury prevention. This information also allows parents and their children to make informed decisions about football participation [28]. The published articles on American football in athletes of high school age and younger were identified by searching Sports Discus (1940–2003), Eric (1967–2003), EMBASE (1988–2003), MEDLINE (1966–2003), CINAHL (1984–2003), and Web of Science (1993–2003).

Two major limitations to cross-investigation comparisons are the definition of what exactly is an injury and what constitutes risk. The numerator refers to the injury events and the denominator reflects the participating players at risk [29, 30]. An epidemiological survey of the literature on high school football injuries [31] revealed numerous methodological problems. Simply put, the calculated injury rate is only good at the identification of cases (numerator) and the identification of the population-at-risk (denominator). Lack of a clear definition of injury, standardized forms, strict record keeping and precise diagnosis results in detection and recall bias. The specific definition of injury is critical, since studies that record all injuries, including minor trauma, can overestimate risk. Injury detection by telephone interview or questionnaire is fraught with inaccuracy. Emergency department chart review may not identify the injured athletes who sought evaluation elsewhere or did not require treatment [32]. Data from insurance files uncovers only the claims-made injuries, which also encourages under-reporting [33]. Parents and coaches may not have the experience to correctly diagnose and report all injuries [23]. Surveys and questionnaires have poor compliance and are fraught with error.

Most published investigations of high school and youth football injuries have not considered the population-at-risk, but have merely reported the number of participants. Injury risk factors cannot be analyzed without simultaneous measurement of injury exposure [34]. The total number of participants used as the denominator fails to account for the time of exposure, which is a key component for a meaningful analysis. Defining the population-at-risk as the players on the team roster at the start of the season does not take into consideration player attrition (transfer bias) or limited playing time (low exposure). Estimation of collective player exposure by calculating the number of players, the number of games and practices, and the approximate length of each practice and games is inaccurate. This method also implies that each practice is the same and each player participates equally in each practice and game.

Football is a noncontinuous participation sport, and interruption of competition between plays makes injury risk assessment according to player-games and player-plays more pragmatic than player-hours. The actual playing time during a 40-minute youth football game (four 10-minute quarters) has been measured at approximately eight minutes [14]. Measurement of exposure to injury by recording the offensive, defensive and special teams' plays is more sensitive. This technique of injury analysis and reporting is similar to tracking the number of bicycle trips or gymnastics maneuvers and should be more accurate in calculating injury rates. Even well-designed studies often use methods of injury incidence calculation that typically do not account for more than one injury per incident or more than one injury per player.

Incidence of Injury

Risk of injury or 'incidence' is determined according to established principles of epidemiological research. Few studies to date have accurately addressed the risk of injury during football game participation, and comparison to other sports or free play is difficult. Participation in competitive football, especially at the youth level, can be difficult for some players and their parents because of a perceived high injury risk. The available literature both supports and refutes this perception.

A prospective study of 6–17-year-old athletes participating in six supervised sports on a military base revealed that football players sustained twice as many orthopedic injuries as any other sport [35]. However, these researchers also found that unsupervised recreational activities contributed twice as many extremity injuries as those occurring during organized sporting events. Baseline injury rate was studied in a cohort of children aged 7–13 participating in community-organized baseball, softball, soccer and football [36]. No differences were detected over a period of two seasons when the injury risk was expressed as injuries per 100 athlete-exposures. Football participation was associated with a higher risk of serious injury (fracture, dislocation, concussion). High school athletes who played football were not at higher risk for injury when compared to students participating in other activities [18]. Junior league organized football was safer than free play based on an analysis of 70 teams [24]. Data collected on athletes in the fourth with grades [14] revealed that the risk of injury in youth football did not appear greater than other recreational or competitive sports. Godshall [37] observed approximately 2,300 Junior League football players over a 17-year period and identified only 2 major injuries. His risk-benefit analysis concluded that the leadership, discipline, self-sacrifice, and sportsmanship learned outweighed the prospect of injury.

On the other hand, surveillance of injuries to high school athletes by athletic trainers revealed that football had the highest injury rate (8.1 per 1,000 athlete-exposures) and volleyball had the lowest (1.7 per 1,000 athlete-exposures) [38]. Another one-year study of 1,283 high school athletes identified 280 injuries with football responsible for 61% [39]. Football was also responsible for the highest percentage (81 injuries/100 participants) of injuries among high school athletes in the Seattle metropolitan area [22], and high school football players were 6 times more likely to have knee surgery compared to the general population [16].

High School

The data on injury rates affecting high school football players are summarized in table 1. Review of table 1 identifies one retrospective study [8] and six prospective [15, 16, 18, 19, 38, 39] studies. Surveys and insurance or emergency record reviews were not included. The study duration ranged from one to nine seasons, although most studies followed the athletes for two to four seasons. Definition of injury varied, but typically included time-lost from participation as one of the criteria. Exposure was measured in only three of the studies by estimating the collective player participation in practices and games. Cross-study comparisons are not reliable if the definition of injury and/or measurement of exposure are inconsistent. Injury rates in the Powell and Barber-Foss [38] and Turbeville [15] studies indicate a range of 13.1–26.4 injuries per 1,000 game exposures and 1.3–5.3 injuries per 1,000 practice exposures. These discrepancies may reflect differences in study design rather than a true difference in injury incidence.

Thompson [31] identified 32 total injuries in 36 players during a single high school football season, but many trivial injuries were likely included.

Table 1. High school football injuries

	Study design	Study duration	Number of injuries/ players	Definition of injury	Measurement of exposure	Data collection method	Injury rate
Moretz [18]	Prospective cohort	Two seasons	241/903	Time lost (altered or lost practice or game)	None (estimated total time at risk)	Player telephone interview	? 0.51 injuries/ player/game hour
Olson [39]	Prospective cohort	Nine seasons	478/1200	Time lost (≥2 practices, ≥1 game)	None	Injury report form	?
Culpepper [8]	Retrospective cohort	Four seasons	1877/?	Treatment sought	None	Clinic record review	?
Prager [19]	Prospective cohort	Four seasons	251/598	Time lost	None	Player or athletic trainer report	?
DeLee [16]	Prospective cohort	One season	2,228/4,399	Any time lost, physician treatment, head injuries	Estimated collective exposure	Athletic trainer report	0.506 injuries/ athlete/year
Powell [38]	Prospective cohort	Three seasons	10,557/?	Time lost (unable to participate in current practice or game), fractures, dental, brain injuries	Collective exposure	Athletic trainer report	26.4 injuries per 1,000 game exposures, 5.3 injuries per 1,000 practice exposures
Turbeville [15]	Prospective cohort Age 12–18	Two seasons	132/717	Time lost (missing a practice/game or alteration of or loss consciousness)	Estimated collective exposure (total number of players × total number of practices and games)	Coach or athletic trainer report	13.1 injuries per 1,000 game exposures, 1.3 injuries per 1,000 practice exposures

Stuart

Turbeville et al. [15] studied injury frequency and risk factors in high school football players. The football coach or an athletic trainer generated an injury report and telephone follow-up confirmed the injury type, location and treatment. Collective exposure was estimated by multiplying the total number of players by the total number of practices and games. Overall risk in this cohort measured 13.1 injuries per 1,000 game exposures and 1.3 injuries per 1,000 practice exposures. Since the actual amount of playing time was not recorded for each player, first-string players were analyzed to indirectly control for playing time. Multivariate analysis revealed that a positive injury history and increasing player experience were the only significant injury predictor variables. The authors concluded that the best predictor of injury was playing experience, not physical characteristics. Injury risk increased 40–60% for every year increase in experience; but experienced players may simply be at higher risk because they participate in more plays during each game.

Youth

Injury rate data for youth football are summarized in table 2 [14, 21, 23, 26]. Surveys and insurance or emergency record reviews were not included. Only four prospective cohort studies were identified. Study duration ranged from one to two seasons and all used a time-loss definition of injury. In the two studies that measured exposure to injury, game injury rates were very similar. Stuart et al. [14] reported 8.5 and Turbeville et al. [23] 8.8 injuries per 1,000 player games respectively. Goldberg [26] gathered injury data by telephone interview and questionnaire on football players aged 9 to 14. The prevalence of injury type and location are somewhat helpful, but no additional conclusions are possible without measurement of exposure time.

The prospective cohort observational analysis by Stuart et al. [14] during a single season showed that youth football injuries are uncommon, occurring once every 8.75 seasons per player. Strengths of this study include a clear definition of injury, standardized forms, strict record keeping and an orthopedic sports medicine physician on site to provide an accurate diagnosis. A coach from each team completed the game participation and exposure form and recorded the total number of offensive and defensive plays, kickoffs and punts for each team. These epidemiological principles foster injury identification with minimal detection and recall bias, along with simultaneous measurement of injury exposure. Overall risk in this cohort was 8.5 injuries per 1,000 player-games and 0.2 injuries per 1,000 player-plays.

Turbeville et al. [23] also reported on injury frequency and risk factors in middle school football players using the same study design as their high school project. First-string players were again studied to indirectly control for playing time. Overall risk in this cohort was 8.8 injuries per 1,000 game exposures, and

Table 2. Youth football injuries

	Study design	Study duration	Number of injuries/players	Definition of injury	Measurement of exposure	Data collection method	Injury rate
Goldberg [26]	Prospective cohort Age 9–14	One season	67/436	Time lost (greater than or equal to one day)	None	Questionnaire completed by league personnel	?
Linder [21]	Prospective cohort Age 11–15	Two seasons	55/340	Time lost (removal from or missing subsequent practice or game)	None	Coach report	?
Stuart [14]	Prospective cohort Age 9–13	One season	55/915	Time lost (remainder of the game), attention of a physician, all concussion, dental, eye and nerve injuries	Individual player game participation, number of plays/game for each team	Physician examination	8.5 injuries per 1,000 player-games, 0.2 injuries per 1,000 player-plays
Turbeville [23]	Prospective cohort Age 10–15	Two seasons	64/646	Time lost (missing practice or game/head injury with impaired consciousness)	Estimated collective exposure (total number of players × total number of practices and games)	Coach or athletic trainer report	8.8 injuries per 1,000 game exposures, 1.0 injuries per 1,000 practice exposures

1.0 injury per 1,000 practice exposures. The incidence of game injury in the youth players is somewhat less than Turbeville et al. [15] reported in high school athletes (13.1 injuries per 1,000 game exposures) using a similar study design.

Player Position
Injuries occur to players who are being tackled, tackling or blocking. Therefore, running backs, lineman and linebackers have the highest injury rate [28]. Injuries causing a time loss of 48 hours were more prevalent for high school offensive players (n = 153) compared to defensive players (n = 98). Excluding specialty teams, high school tackles and linebackers sustained the most injuries based on a percentage of total injuries. No exposure data for players or positions was recorded [19]. Youth football running backs and lineman were at highest risk for injuries, especially to the knee [14, 23].

Injury Characteristics

Injury Onset
The overwhelming majority of injuries in both high school and youth football are sudden or acute. Little information is available on the incidence and mechanism of overuse injuries in these young athletes.

Injury Location
Injury location expressed as a percentage of total injuries is summarized for high school football studies in table 3 [8, 15, 16, 18, 38, 39] and for youth football studies in table 4 [14, 23, 24, 26]. A review of table 3 indicated that the lower extremity is the most frequently injured body region (31–59%) followed by the upper extremity (21–34%). The knee (15–37%) and ankle (11–27%) joints are most susceptible to football trauma. Upper extremity injuries typically involve the shoulder (8–15%), and wrist and hand (7–11%). Table 4 shows a similar distribution for youth players with the majority involving the lower extremity (36–51%) followed by the upper extremity (25–41%). The knee (17–22%) and ankle (10–17%) are again most susceptible for the lower extremity, the wrist and hand (14–30%) for the upper extremity. The ankle physes (distal tibial and fibular growth plates) are especially vulnerable for a fracture in skeletally immature athletes [14].

Although cervical spine injuries are uncommon in most studies, a preseason examination of 104 high school football players revealed a history of neck injury in 17, positive physical examination findings in 2 players, and radiographic abnormalities in 8 [40]. Seventy-four high school players were studied over two seasons in an attempt to identify all injuries to the cervical

Table 3. High school injury location

Percentage of total injuries	Olson [39] n = 478	Moretz [18] n = 241	Culpepper [8] n = 1,877	DeLee [16] n = 2,228	Powell [38] n = 10,557	Turbeville [15] n = 132	Range
Head			8	5		7	
Neck	10	6		1	13	2	6–15
Face				4	2	6	
Back	2	5	5	8		4	2–8
Trunk	5		3	1	9	1	1–9
Upper extremity	26	21	34	23	26	22	21–34
Shoulder	9	7	13	11		9	7–11
Upper arm	1		1		12	2	1–2
Lower arm	1	<1	2				1–2
Elbow	2	3	3	4			2–4
Wrist			3		14	3	8–15
Hand	13	10	12	8		5	1–3
Pelvis/groin			<1			3	2–17
Hip		12	2	7	17		31–50
Lower extremity	58	58	46	48	31	59	4–10
Upper leg	4	4	5			10	4–10
Lower leg	4		4	8			4–8
Knee	37	22	22	20	15	20	15–37
Ankle			11	18		27	11–27
Foot	12	22	4	2	16	2	2–4
Other	1	10	<1				

spine. Eight neck injuries were documented, including six muscle strains, one 'stinger', and one transient neurapraxia.

Situation

The risk of injury appears to be greater in competition than in practice, both at the high school and youth levels. High school football injuries are much more common in games than in practice [15, 16, 18, 40]. Moretz et al. [18] found the risk of injury for Oklahoma high school football players to be 18 times higher in a game that is a practice. The risk of injury in youth football is also higher in games, but injury incidence appears less than high school reports [14, 23]. Inconsistency in exposure measurement techniques and different expressions of injury rate make comparison of the available research difficult. Turbeville et al. [15, 23] reported a 10-fold increased risk of game injury (13.1 injuries per 1,000 game exposures) than in practice (1.3 injuries per 1,000 practice exposures)

Table 4. Youth injury location

Percentage of total injuries	Roser [24] n = 48	Goldberg [26] n = 67	Stuart [14] n = 55	Turbeville [23] n = 64	Range
Head	8	10	7	2	2–10
Face					
Neck					
Back	5	3	9	9	3–9
Trunk	6	5	5	6	5–6
Upper extremity		32	25	41	25–41
Shoulder	2	5	7		5–7
Upper arm					
Elbow	1	6	4	11	4–6
Lower arm					
Wrist	7		9	17	14–30
Hand	9	21	5	13	5–13
Pelvis/groin			2	3	2–3
Hip		3			3
Lower extremity		47	51	36	36–51
Upper leg			5		2–10
Lower leg			5	2	
Knee	8	22	20	17	17–22
Ankle		10	15	17	10–17
Foot		15	4		4–15
Other			2		

in high school players and almost 9-fold increased risk of game injury (8.8 injuries per 1,000 game exposures) than in practice (1.0 injury per 1,000 practice exposures) in youth players.

Chronometry

The risk of injury was 510 per 1,000 player-game-hours of exposure compared to 150 per 1,000 player-practice-hours during the preseason and 28 per 1,000 player-practice-hours during the season [18]. These rates suggest that injuries are 5.4 times more likely in preseason practice and 18.2 times more likely in games than in inseason practice.

Injury Severity

Most youth football injuries are mild, and the most common type is a contusion. Severity of injury is typically based on time loss until return to participation.

Table 5. High school injury type

Perncetage of total injuries	Moretz [18]	Olson [39]	Culpepper [8]	DeLee [16]	Powell [38]	Turbeville [15]
Sprain	40	21	32	45	32	54
Strain	22		12		21	
Contusion	18	14	25	21		17
Fracture	13	24	11	7	8	11
Dislocation		8	2	3		5
Concussion		9	1	5		6
Laceration			<1	16		1
Dental				2		
Other	7	37	16		39	6

Table 6. Youth injury type

Percentage of total injuries	Roser [24]	Goldberg [26]	Linder [21]	Stuart [14]	Turbeville [23]
Sprain	35	34	45	9	55
Strain		12		20	
Contusion	17	22	33	60	17
Fracture	35	15	18	7	27
Dislocation	1	4			
Concussion	4	6		2	
Laceration	7		4		2
Abrasion		2			
Dental					
Other		2		2	

An example of severity grading includes: mild (no limitations expected and either no time loss or players expected back at football within 3 days); moderate (athletes returned within 4–14 days); and severe (long-term sequelae expected and athletes expected to be out of football longer than 14 days).

Injury Types

Type of injury is summarized for high school players in table 5 [8, 15, 16, 18, 38, 39] and youth players in table 6 [14, 21, 23, 24, 26]. Most studies agree that minor injuries such as contusions, strains and sprains account for the bulk of all injuries. Turbeville et al. [15] showed that sprains and strains were most common in high school players, followed by contusions, and fractures. Injury type is very similar in high school and youth players, but the diagnostic terminology is not uniform. Sprains (9–45%) and strains (12–22%) combined account for approximately half of all injuries at both levels. Contusions represent between 14 and 60% and concussions only 1–9% of all injuries. Fractures occur in 7–24% of injuries to high school players and 7–35% of injuries to youth players. These fractures typically involve the growth plates of the wrist and ankle.

Catastrophic Injury

The likelihood of serious or catastrophic injury to youth football players is relatively small, but the risk increases for high school players. Mueller [41] defined catastrophic injury as any severe injury incurred during participation in a school-sponsored sport. These injuries are categorized as fatal, nonfatal (permanent or severe functional disability) or serious (no permanent functional disability, but severe injury). Sports injuries were further classified as direct or indirect. Direct injuries result from participation in the skills of the sport. Indirect injuries are caused by systemic failure as a result of exertion while participating in a sport activity or by complication secondary to a nonfatal injury.

Fatalities

The Annual Survey of Football Injury Research conducted by Mueller [42] registered 684 total football fatalities at all levels of play from 1945 through 1994. Most of the head injury fatalities (n = 345, 74.2%) and cervical spine fatalities (n = 76, 65.5%) occurred to high school players during games. The total number of fatalities climbed to 712 through 1999 [41]. Head injuries were responsible for 491 (69%), cervical spine injuries for 116 (16.3%), and other injuries for 105 (14.7%).

Football head-related fatalities were most prevalent in junior and senior high school (75%) largely due to the number of participants. The volume of high school players was estimated at 1.5 million as compared to 75,000 college players. Fatal head injuries usually occurred while tackling or being tackled during a game. Subdural hematoma was the most common diagnosis (75%). The declining rate of football head-related fatalities is likely due to the 1976 rule change prohibiting initial contact with the head or face together with improved coaching of blocking and tackling techniques.

Cantu and Mueller [43] identified catastrophic American football head and spine injuries to high school, college, sandlot and professional players by analyzing epidemiological and medical data from 1977–1998. Catastrophic injuries were defined as death, brain or spinal cord injury, and cranial or spinal fracture. During this 11-year period, 118 football players died, 200 received a permanent spinal cord injury, and 66 suffered a permanent cerebral injury. Although the data were not broken down by age or level, 164 of the 200 cervical cord injuries were sustained by high school players and all 66 cerebral injuries occurred at the high school or college level.

Concussion

Despite the available data, most parents are uninformed about the risks of severe brain injury from their children playing high school football [44]. Athletic trainers recorded injury and exposure data for varsity athletes in 10 different sports at 235 high schools in a 1-year study [45]. Mild traumatic brain injury was diagnosed in 1,219 participants during the 3-year study period. Football accounted for 63.4 percent of the head injuries. Six cases of subdural hematoma and intracranial injury were identified in football players. Head injury rates were 11 times higher for games than for practice [46].

The incidence of concussion, common signs and symptoms as well as return-to-play criteria were analyzed from a survey of high school and collegiate football team athletic trainers [47]. Players who sustained a concussion were 3 times more likely to sustain a second concussion in the same season compared with uninjured players. Only 9% of concussed athletes lost consciousness, 86% developed a headache, and 31% returned to play on the same day. These observations are important, though based on a survey with a 62% response rate. Players, coaches and health care providers should be aware of the increased risk of a second concussion, and symptomatic athletes should never be allow to return to play.

Concussion appears to be relatively uncommon in youth football players [14, 24, 26]. Stuart et al. [14] recorded only one concussion when over 900 youth players aged 9–13 years were carefully followed during a single season. Turbeville et al. [23] identified only one mild head injury during a two-season study of middle school athletes.

Injury Risk Factors

Risk factors for injury can be intrinsic (personal), which represent characteristics of the specific player, or extrinsic (environment, equipment), from features out of the athlete's control (table 7). Determination of a true cause and effect relationship is very difficult because of numerous confounding variables. Increasing age and level of play appear to be associated with increase in injury incidence, but the relationship of body weight to injury risk remains unclear.

Table 7. Injury risk factors

Intrinsic	Extrinsic
Age	Conditioning
Grade in school	Field conditions
Tanner stage	Helmet type
Weight	Shoulder pad type
Body fat	Shoe type
Ligamentous laxity	Knee braces
Playing experience	
Psychosocial factors	
Dangerous activities	

Intrinsic Factors
Physical

Goldberg et al. [26] could not identify a correlation between injury risk and age in youth football players. However, Stuart et al. [14] found that the risk of injury to youth football players increased with level of play (grade in school) and player age. The risk of injury for an eighth grade player was 4 times greater than the risk of injury for a fourth grade player. Potential contributing factors included increased size, strength, speed, and aggressiveness.

Linder et al. [21] examined the relationship between sexual maturity (Tanner stage) and the incidence of injury in junior high school football players. The coach recorded an injury if a player was removed from a practice or a game. An overall injury rate of 16% was reported over two seasons. No serious or permanently disabling injuries occurred. Ten fractures, including five physeal injuries were diagnosed. Injuries were more prevalent in the older players who were also more physically mature (Tanner stages 3, 4, 5). The authors admit that no direct conclusions can be drawn since individual exposure data were not collected.

Turbeville et al. [15] found that injured players were older, bigger, stronger, more experienced, and more likely to have sustained an injury in the previous season. The increased injury risk to the more experienced than uninjured players may actually reflect increased playing time, aggressiveness, or pubescence.

The North Carolina Study investigated junior and senior high school football injuries and also measured grip strength, physiologic maturation, ponderal index (weight relative to height), age, height, weight and body fat (subscapular skinfold) in 466 athletes. [48] Junior high players were less likely to be injured even though both levels had a wide variation in sexual maturation. The injured junior high players were lighter and less mature than noninjured teammates. In the author's opinion, 17% of all injuries were preventable, resulting from poor equipment, hazardous conditions or improper technique.

Tanner's method of assessing sexual maturity was used in 340 male football players between the ages of 11 and 15 [21]. Each team's coach recorded injuries over two seasons if a player was removed from a practice or game and/or missed a subsequent practice or game. Tanner stages 5, 4, and 3 combined were associated with more injuries than Tanner stages 2 and 1 combined. Higher injury prevalence was evident with increasing age in these adolescent athletes. Player age was not controlled when testing for maturity as a risk factor. No exposure data were recorded, and the authors admit that the more mature athletes may have received more playing time. This study suggests that increasing sexual maturity may be a risk factor for adolescent football injuries.

Stuart et al. [14] compared the risk of injury for players above and below the mean body weight according to each grade level. A trend was evident that heavier players (individual body weight $>$ mean body weight) sustained more injuries than lighter players (individual body weight $<$ mean body weight). However, discriminate function analyses with weight predicting injury revealed no significant relationship between body weight and injury.

A prospective cohort analysis of 216 high school football players was designed to determine adiposity is associated with increased risk of injury. Athletic trainers recorded injuries as well as practice and game exposure time. Skinfold measurements revealed body fat range of 9.3–40.2%. Eighty-six injuries occurred during 15,207 hours of total playing time for an injury rate of 0.026 injuries/player/1,000 hours. The trend was for players with more body fat, greater body weight, and greater body mass index to sustain lower extremity injuries. Body mass index greater than $26 \, kg/m^2$ was consistently (except $>34 \, kg/m^2$) associated with risk of lower extremity injury ($p < 0.05$) [49].

Preseason height, weight, and triceps/subscapular skinfold were measured in 98 high school football players. During the season, certified athletic trainers recorded all injuries that required one of these players to miss at least one practice or game. Twenty-seven players (28%) had the sum of skinfolds $\geq$95th percentile for age, but the overall prevalence was not significantly elevated when compared to player's $\leq$95th percentile. Although this study did not show an increased injury risk for obese football players, the high incidence of obesity in this athletic population was alarming [50].

No correlation was found between generalized ligamentous laxity and risk of knee or ankle ligament injury in 402 high school football players followed during a single season [51]. An abnormal preseason history or physical exam did not predict an increased risk of neck injury in these high school athletes [52].

Psychosocial
An investigation to test the relationship of anger/aggression, attention and stressful life events to injury and to determine whether the relationship of

stressful events to injury is mediated by anger or by impaired vigilant or focused attention [53]. High school football players completed preseason measures of anger, vigilant attention or focused attention, and stressful life events and were then followed through one season to identify injuries. Logistic regression indicated that high anger directed outward ($p < 0.05$) and low focused attention ($p < 0.01$) increased injury risk, while stressful life events and vigilant attention interacted. Injury risk was elevated when recent stress was present ($p < 0.05$) and increased as vigilance decreased, suggesting that stressful life events elevate injury risk by reducing vigilance.

Using the Life Event Scale for Adolescents, Coddington and Troxell [54] postulated that a player's mental or emotional state might increase the risk of injury. They based this opinion on the fact that high school players, who experienced more family instability, parental illness, separations, divorces and deaths were more likely to sustain a significant injury. Their review of coaches' records identified only 23 injuries. This small sample size and other possible confounding variables do not allow for a definite association between the player's emotions and risk factor of injury.

Dangerous Activities

'Spearing' involves flexing the neck and initiating contact with the top of the helmet. This dangerous manoeouvre has been associated with cervical spine fracture/dislocation and spinal cord injury. As a result, physicians, administrators and coaches preached avoidance of using the head as the primary point of contact in tackling and blocking. In January 1996, the National Alliance Football Rules Committee changed the rules to make 'butt-blocking' or 'face-tackling' a personal foul (15-yard penalty). Coaches need to teach proper blocking and tackling techniques, which do not involve using the facemask or top of the helmet as the primary point of contact [55]

Despite these concerns, a survey of Louisiana high school football players identified an alarming rate of players who admitted to tackling with the top of their helmet. Eighty-three percent of those players stated that their coach taught these dangerous techniques [56].

A survey of Minnesota high school football coaches raised some concerns about players using illegal techniques such as butt blocking and face tackling [57].

Heck [58] reviewed 9 game films from a high school football season to establish the cumulative incidence per season of ball carrier spearing and concurrent defensive spearing by tacklers. During a single season, 167 incidents of ball carrier spearing (1 per 5.2 plays) and 72 incidents of concurrent defensive spearing (1 per 2.3 ball carrier spears) were identified. Despite the frequency of these rule violations, the game officials did not call any spearing penalties. The authors encourage officials to acknowledge these rule infractions and ask coaches to teach correct ball carrying, blocking and tackling techniques. Lack of rules enforcement is a modifiable risk factor for injury.

Extrinsic Factors

Training Methods or Conditions

Cahill et al. [59] compared the circumstances, number and severity of knee injuries during a 4-year period when football players participated in a preseason-conditioning program to the previous 4 years where no such program existed. The 5–6 week total body conditioning program included cardiovascular exercise, heat acclimatization, weight training, flexibility drills and agility exercises. The knee injury rate per 1,000 athletes was 68 for the no conditioning group and approximately 40 for the closely-supervised conditioning group. The operative rate per 1,000 players was 15.2 for the no conditioning group, 5.7 for the closely-supervised conditioning group and 2.3 for the less-supervised conditioning group. Early season knee injuries were reduced by 67% in the conditioning groups as compared to the no conditioning group. The authors concluded that preseason conditioning significantly reduces the early season knee injuries, the total number of knee injuries and the injury severity.

Environment

Wisconsin high school football teams were studied to determine the association of injury to field conditions [60]. 'Good' conditions were associated with the highest frequency of injury (3.3 injuries/game). 'Wet' and 'slippery' conditions were associated with the lowest rate (1.8 injuries/game). 'Hard' and 'muddy' conditions were associated with intermediate injury risk (2.3 and 2.1 injuries/game respectively). The authors postulated that wet and slippery conditions caused a reduction in player velocity and rotational stability of the shoe with the ground.

Adkison et al. [61] reported on 349 time-loss injuries from 424 high school football games played on natural grass and 236 games played on synthetic turf. Data analyses showed the injury rate for Astroturf (0.63 injuries per game) as compared to grass (0.51 injuries per game) and Tartan Turf (0.28 injuries per game). A prospective study of 26 high school football teams during 148 games played on grass and 80 games played on artificial turf revealed higher injury rate and severity on the synthetic surface [62]. The artificial turf studied was a single stadium where 12 of the schools played a majority of their games. The higher injury rates for the synthetic surface were predominantly sustained when the turf was dry, implicating increased traction as a potential risk factor.

The risk of knee and ankle injuries was reduced by 30% with resurfaced fields and regular cleats, and by 46% with resurfaced fields and soccer shoes when compared to schools with no changes.

Equipment

Mueller and Blyth [63] reported on football injuries in 43 North Carolina high schools. Investigators visited each school during the preseason to evaluate the protective equipment of each player for make, fit and condition. The investigators then returned to the schools each week to interview each injured player. The North Carolina High School Football Injury Study suggested that specific brand name football helmets and shoulder pads were associated with higher injury 'rates', and a properly maintained playing surface combined with soccer-style shoes reduced knee and ankle injures. The data provided are actually the prevalence of injury according to specific equipment brand. However, the author's conclusions are difficult to substantiate, since no exposure data were provided.

The relationship of football shoe design and injury rate encouraged regulations on the size and configuration of cleats. The conventional shoe, with seven $3/4 \times 3/8$ inch cleats, was associated with a higher incidence and severity of injury when compared to the soccer-style shoe with fourteen $3/8 \times 1/2$ inch cleats [64]. Four different football shoe cleat types were prospectively evaluated in high school football players to determine torsional resistance and the relationship with anterior cruciate ligament tears [65]. The edge design with longer, irregular cleats placed at the peripheral margin of the sole produced significantly higher torsional resistance and was associated with a significantly higher anterior cruciate ligament injury rate when compared to the flat, screw-in, and pivot disc designs.

Deppen and Landfried [66] compared high school football players at schools with mandatory or voluntary prophylactic knee brace use by tracking injuries, practice and game exposure. They found no differences in knee injury risk with and without bracing.

Suggestions for Injury Prevention

Youth and high school football injury risk may be reduced by player conditioning and strength training, the use of high quality, well-fit equipment, coaching of safety fundamentals, avoidance of dangerous activities, enforcement of existing rules, as well as proper medical supervision and care.

The 1976 rule change prohibiting initial contact with the head or face (spearing, face tackling and butt blocking) together with improved coaching of blocking and tackling techniques appears to have reduced the incidence of head and neck injuries. This rule change has also played a very important role in the decline of football fatalities. Head and cervical spine trauma resulting in football-related fatalities are depicted by decade from 1945 through 1994 in figure 1. The

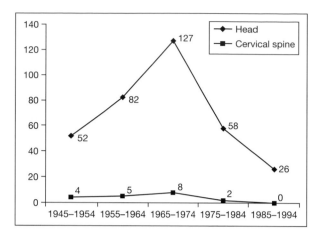

Fig. 1. High school football fatalities [45].

incidence of high school football fatalities over time is depicted in figure 2. Mueller [41, 42] recommended additional measures to reduce head and neck fatalities:

- mandatory medical examinations for all football athletes
- education of players, parents and coaches
- coaching of proper blocking and tackling techniques
- strengthening of the neck muscles
- strict enforcement of rules
- physician or athletic trainer coverage
- preparedness for all emergencies
- immediate medical attention for any player with signs of head trauma

Injury prevention or 'acceptable risk' can be achieved by minimizing extrinsic risk factors and counterbalancing intrinsic risk factors. Intrinsic factors include the developmental mindset along with biologic characteristics of the individual. Extrinsic factors include predictors of injury related to the activity or environment. In reality, the literature contains a paucity of actual preventative trials.

A cohort interventional analysis by Bixler and Jones [67] attempted to determine whether a warm-up and stretching session at half-time affected injury risk in the 3rd quarter of the game. The authors found a significant decrease in 3rd quarter sprains and strains, but no difference in total injuries. Preassignment of participating teams may have introduced bias since increased susceptibility by an individual team or a particular game may have skewed the results.

Neck circumference and range of motion were studied in 40 high school football players [68]. No correlation was found between the athlete's neck size and range of motion. The authors speculate that proper fitting equipment, neck conditioning exercises and changes in the rules might reduce the risk of injury to the cervical spine region in football players. Although impingement of the helmet and facemask against the shoulder pads may restrict motion and tensile forces, the most dangerous mechanism of injury is an axial load to the partially flexed cervical spine.

Observations of high school football players over a 12-year period by Cahill and Griffith [6] suggested that a preseason conditioning program, consisting of cardiovascular stress, heat acclimatization, weight training, flexibility drills and agility exercises, reduced the number and severity of knee injuries. A follow-up study showed that a decrease in supervision of the quality of the preseason program did not affect the apparent benefits [59]. No exposure data were collected, and no other potential confounding variables were examined.

Despite the lack of true epidemiological research, the experiences of numerous authors provides some important recommendations that may prevent injuries or improve the care of the athlete:

- provide emergency medical services (physicians, athletic trainers, para-medics or emergency medical technicians) during games [69]
- match players by Tanner stage and development [70]
- encourage appropriate training and conditioning [70]
- properly fit equipment and footwear [70]
- educate coaches and parents [70]
- maintain playing fields [17]
- use of soccer-style shoes [17]
- allow only noncontact and controlled activities in practice [17, 63]
- increase vigilance over technique during injury-prone preseason practices [17]
- delay return to full contact until complete recovery of injured players [63]
- teach fundamental blocking and tackling skills [39]
- strengthen the neck muscles [39]
- ensure qualified coaches to render emergency care prior to physician evaluation or emergency transport [39]
- forbid use of the head for initial contact [39]

In Garrick's opinion, no new items of equipment would significantly reduce football injuries [71].

According to the FIMS/WHO Ad Hoc Committee on Sports and Children, sport governing bodies should: monitor the level of intensity and categories of competition in their sports, prepare and maintain ongoing statistics of illness and injury, certify the credentials of coaches and determine standards for protective equipment, playing fields, and duration of competition.

Suggestions for Further Research

To make informed decisions about football injury prevention, risk must be reliably identified in relation to multiple variables. Comparison of injury incidence and risk factors requires well-designed injury epidemiology studies. Ideally, protocols involve the prospective analysis of a defined cohort by an experienced research team. Each study needs a standardized, strict definition of injury and medical terminology, diagnosis by a sports medicine professional, accurate measurement of player exposure, and data analysis based on injury per player play. Longer study duration may determine residual injury effects and cost. High quality epidemiology study design will allow assessment of numerous variables such as player size, rules, protective equipment and playing surface.

Football head-related fatalities, concussion, neck and spinal cord injuries have been reduced by rule changes and improved coaching of blocking and tackling techniques. An increased emphasis on research to test the efficacy of these and other preventative measures is needed.

Youth football leagues are typically organized by age or grade level with some position restrictions according to body weight. A better understanding of the association between injury risk and player age, physical maturity and body weight may promote prevention through validated matching strategies.

Acknowledgment

The author thanks Patricia J. Erwin of the Mayo Medical Library for her assistance with the literature review.

References

1   Landry GL: Sports injuries in childhood. Pediatr Ann 1992;21:165–168.
2   Gallagher SS, Finison K, Guyer B, Goodenough S: The incidence of injuries among 87,000 Massachusetts children and adolescents: Results of the 1980–1981 statewide childhood injury prevention program surveillance system. Am J Public Health 1984;74:1340–1347.
3   Mueller FO, Blyth CS: Can we continue to improve injury statistics in football? Phys Sportsmed 1984;12:79–83.
4   Hutchinson MR, Nasser R: Common sports injuries in children and adolescents. Medscape General Medicine 2000;2:http://www.medscape.com/viewarticle/408524.

5   Mueller FO, Blyth CS: Football injury update – 1979 season. Improved conditioning, rule changes, and a helmet standard helped reduce football fatalities to an all-time low in 1979. Phys Sportsmed 1980;8:53–55.

6   Cahill BR, Griffith EH: Effect of preseason conditioning on the incidence and severity of high school football knee injuries. Am J Sports Med 1978;6:180–184.

7   Mueller FO, Blyth CS: An update on football deaths and catastrophic injuries. Phys Sportsmed 1986;14:139–42.

8   Culpepper MI, Niemann KMW: A comparison of game and practice injuries in high school football. Phys Sportsmed 1983;11:117–122.

9   Maroon JC, Steele PB, Berlin R: Football head and neck injuries – an update. Clin Neurosurg 1980;27:414–429.

10 Mueller FO, Blyth CS, Cantu RC: Catastrophic spine injuries in football. Phys Sportsmed 1989;17.

11 Dagiau RF, Dillman CJ, Milner EK: Relationship between exposure time and injury in football. Am J Sports Med 1980;8:257–260.

12 Lackland DT, Akers P, Hirata I Jr: High school football injuries in South Carolina: A computerized survey. JSC Med Assoc 1982;78:75–78.

13 Stocker BD, Nyland JA, Caborn DN, Sternes R, Ray JM: Results of the Kentucky high school football knee injury survey. J K Med Assoc 1997;95:458–464.

14 Stuart MJ, Morrey MA, Smith AM, Meis JK, Ortiguera CJ: Injuries in youth football: A prospective observational cohort analysis among players aged 9 to 13 years.[erratum appears in Mayo Clin Proc 2003 Jan;78:120.] Mayo Clin Proc 2002;77:317–322.

15 Turbeville SD, Cowan LD, Owen WL, Asal NR, Anderson MA: Risk factors for injury in high school football players. Am J Sports Med 2003;31:974–980.

16 DeLee JC, Farney WC: Incidence of injury in Texas high school football. Am J Sports Med 1992;20:575–580.

17 Halpern B, Thompson N, Curl WW, Andrews JR, Hunter SC, and Boring JR: High school football injuries: Identifying the risk factors. (Les lesions consecutives a la pratique du football americain scolaire: identification des facteurs de risque.) Am J Sports Med 1987;15:316–320.

18 Moretz A 3rd, Rashkin A, Grana WA: Oklahoma high school football injury study: A preliminary report. J Okla State Med Assoc 1978;71:85–88

19 Prager BI, Fitton WL, Cahill BR, Olson GH: High school football injuries: A prospective study and pitfalls of data collection. Am J Sports Med 1989;17:681–685.

20 Thompson N, Halpern B, Curl WW, Andrews JR, Hunter SC, Boring JR 3rd, McLeod WD: High school football injuries: Evaluation.[erratum appears in Am J Sports Med 1987 May–Jun;15:257.] Am J Sports Med 1987;15:117–124.

21 Linder MM, Townsend DJ, Jones JC, Balkcom IL, Anthony CR: Incidence of adolescent injuries in junior high school football and its relationship to sexual maturity. Clin J Sport Med 1995;5:167–170.

22 Garrick JG, Requa, RK: Injuries in high school sports. Pediatrics 1978;61:465–469.

23 Turbeville SD, Cowan LD, Asal NR, Owen WL, Anderson MA: Risk factors for injury in middle school football players. Am J Sports Med 2003;31:276–281.

24 Roser LA, Clawson DK: Football injuries in the very young athlete. Clin Orthop 1970;69:219–223.

25 Godshall RW: Junior league football: Risks versus benefits. J Sports Med 1975;3:139–144.

26 Goldberg B, Rosenthal PP, Nicholas JA: Injuries in youth football. Phys Sportsmed 1984;12:122–130.

27 Robey JM, Blyth CS, Mueller FO: Athletic injuries: Application of epidemiology methods. J Am Med Assoc 1971;217:184–189.

28 Porter CD: Football injuries. Phys Med Rehab Clin N Am 1999;10:95–115.

29 Wallace RB: Application of epidemiologic principles to sports injury research. Public Health Report 1985;100:586–588.

30 Noyes FR, Lindenfeld TN, Marshall MT: What determines an athletic injury (definition)? Who determines an injury (occurrence)? Am J Sports Med 1987;5:595–568.

31 Thompson RR: A study of the type and cost of football injuries. A single season in a Minnesota high school. Minn Med 1986;69:656–658.

32 Zoch TW, Cleveland DA, McCormick J, Toyama K, Nordstrom DL: Football injuries in a rural area. Wis Med J 1996;95:570–573.

33   Pritchett JW: A claims-made study of knee injuries due to football in high school athletes. J Pediatr Orthop 1988;8:551–553.

34   Langburt W, Cohen B, Akhthar N, O'Neill K, Lee JC: Incidence of concussion in high school football players of Ohio and Pennsylvania. J Child Neurol 2001;16:83–85.

35   Chambers RB: Orthopaedic injuries in athletes (ages 6 to 17). Comparison of injuries occurring in six sports. Am J Sports Med 1979;7:195–197.

36   Radelet MA, Lephart SM, Rubinstein EN, Myers JB: Survey of the injury rate for children in community sports. Pediatrics 2002;110:1–11.

37   Godshall RW: Junior League Football: Risks versus benefits. Primary Care; Clinics in Office Practice 7:331–341.

38   Powell JW, Barber-Foss KD: Injury patterns in selected high school sports: A review of the 1995–1997 seasons. J Athl Train 1999;34:277–284.

39   Olson OC: Spokane study: High school football injuries. Phys Sportsmed 1979;7:75–82.

40   Albright JP, Moses JM, Feldick HG, Dolan KD, Burmeister LF: Nonfatal cervical spine injuries in interscholastic football. J Am Med Assoc 1976;236:1243–1245.

41   Mueller FO: Catastrophic head injuries in high school and collegiate sports. J Athl Train 2001;36: 312–315.

42   Mueller FO: Fatalities from head and cervical spine injuries occurring in tackle football: 50 years' experience. Clin Sports Med 1998;17:169–181.

43   Cantu RC, Mueller FO: Catastrophic football injuries: 1977–1998. Neurosurgery 2000;47: 673–675; discussion 675–677.

44   Goldhaber GM: A national survey about parent awareness of the risk of severe brain injury from playing football. J Athl Train 1993;28: 306–311.

45   McLain LG, Reynolds S: Sports injuries in a high school. Pediatrics 1989;84:446–450.

46   Powell JW, Barber-Foss KD: Traumatic brain injury in high school athletes.[comment]. J Am Med Assoc 1999;282:958–963.

47   Guskiewicz KM, Weaver NL, Padua DA, Garrett WE Jr: Epidemiology of concussion in collegiate and high school football players. Am J Sports Med 2000;28:643–650.

48   Mueller F, Blyth C: Epidemiology of sports injuries in children. Clin Sports Med 1982;1:343–352.

49   Gomez JE, Ross SK, Calmbach WL, Kimmel RB, Schmidt DR, Dhanda R: Body fatness and increased injury rates in high school football linemen. Clin J Sport Med 1998;8:115–120.

50   Kaplan TA, Digel SL, Scavo VA, Arellana SB: Effect of obesity on injury risk in high school football players. Clin J Sport Med 1995;5:43–7.

51   Clark JL, Challop RS, McCabe EB: Predicting lower extremity injuries in high school football players. J Am Med Assoc 1971;217:1552–1553.

52   Marzo JM, Simmons EH, Whieldon TJ: Neck injuries to high school football players in Western New York State. NY State J Med 1991;91:46–49.

53   Thompson NJ, Morris RD: Predicting injury risk in adolescent players: The importance of psychological variables. J Pediatr Psychol 1994;19:415–429.

54   Coddington RD, Troxell JR: Effect of emotional factors on football injury rates – A pilot-study. J Human Stress 1980;6:3–5.

55   Cooper DL: High school football injuries. (editorial). South Med J 1976;69:1257.

56   Lawrence DW, Stewart GW, Christy DM, Gibbs LI, Ouellette M: High school football-related cervical spinal cord injuries in Louisiana: The athlete's perspective. J L State Med Soc 1997;149: 27–31.

57   Gerberich SG, Priest JD, Boen JR, Straub CP, Maxwell RE: Concussion incidences and severity in secondary school varsity football players. Am J Public Health 1983;73:1370–1375.

58   Heck JF: The incidence of spearing by ball carriers and their tacklers during a high school football season; in Hoerner EF (ed): Head and Neck Injuries in Sports. Philadelphia, American Society for Testing & Materials, 1994, pp 239–249.

59   Cahill BR, Griffith EH, Sunderlin J, Madden T, Weltman A: Effect of preseason conditioning. High school football knee injuries. IMJ Ill Med J 1984;166:356–358.

60   Andresen BL, Hoffman MD, Barton LW: High school football injuries: Field conditions and other factors. Wis Med J 1989;88:28–31.

61   Adkison JW, Requa RK, Garrick JG: Injury rates in high school football. A comparison of synthetic surfaces and grass fields. Clin Orthop 1974;99:131–136.

62 Bramwell ST, Garrick JG, Requa RK: High school football injuries: A pilot comparison of playing surfaces. Med Sci Sports 1972;4:166–169.
63 Mueller FD, Blyth CS: North Carolina high school football injury study: Equipment and prevention. J Sportsmed 1974;2:1–10.
64 Torg JS, Quedenfeld T: Effect of shoe type and cleat length on incidence and severity of knee injuries among high school football players. Res Q 1971;42:203–211.
65 Lambson RB, Barnhill BS, Higgins RW: Football cleat design and its effect on anterior cruciate ligament injuries: A three-year prospective study. Am J Sports Med 1996;24:155–159.
66 Deppen RJ, Landfried MJ: Efficacy of prophylactic knee bracing in high school football players. J Orthop Sports Phys Ther 1994;20:243–246.
67 Bixler B, Jones RL: High-school football injuries: Effects of a post-halftime warm-up and stretching routine. Fam Pract Res J 1992;12:131–139.
68 Pearl AJ, Mayer PW: Neck motion in the high school football player. Am J Sports Med 1979;7:231–233.
69 Silverstein BM: Injuries in youth league football. Phys Sportsmed 1979;7:105–108;111.
70 Rome ES: Sports-related injuries among adolescents: When do they occur, and how can we prevent them? Pediatr Rev 1995;16:184–187; quiz 188.
71 Garrick, JG: The facts about school athletic injuries – A conversation with Dr. James Garrick. NASSP Bulletin 1981;65:43–49.

Michael J. Stuart, MD
Mayo Clinic, 200 First Street SW
Rochester MN 55905 (USA)
Tel. +1 507 284 3462, Fax +1 507 284 5539, E-Mail stuart.michael@mayo.edu

Maffulli N, Caine DJ (eds): Epidemiology of Pediatric Sports Injuries: Team Sports.
Med Sport Sci. Basel, Karger, 2005, vol 49, pp 86–119

....

Ice Hockey Injuries

Brian W. Benson, Willem H. Meeuwisse

Faculty of Kinesiology, Sport Medicine Centre and
Department of Community Health Sciences,
Faculty of Medicine, University of Calgary, Calgary, Alberta, Canada

Abstract

Objective: This article reviews the distribution and determinants of injuries reported in the pediatric ice hockey literature, and suggests potential injury prevention strategies and directions for further research. **Data Sources:** Thirteen electronic databases, the ISI Web of Science, and 'grey literature' databases were searched using a combination of Medical Subject Headings and text words to identify potentially relevant articles. The bibliographies of selected studies were searched to identify additional articles. Studies were selected for review based on predetermined inclusion and exclusion criteria. **Main Results:** A comparison between studies on this topic area was difficult due to the variability in research designs, definition of injury, study populations, and measurements used to assess injury. The majority of injuries were sustained during games compared with practices. The two most commonly reported injuries were sprains/strains and contusions. Players competing at the Minor hockey, High School, and Junior levels of competition sustained most of their injuries to the upper extremity, head, and lower extremity, respectively. The primary mechanism of injury was body checking, followed by stick and puck contact. The frequency of catastrophic eye injuries has been significantly reduced with the world-wide mandation of full facial protection for all Minor hockey players. **Conclusions:** Specific hockey-related injury risk factors are poorly delineated and rarely studied among pediatric ice hockey players leaving large gaps in the knowledge of appropriate prevention strategies. Risk management strategies should be focused at avoiding unnecessary foreseeable risk, and controlling the risks inherent to the sport. Suggestions for injury prevention and future research are discussed.

Introduction

Ice hockey is one of Canada's most popular sports, with more than 500,000 registered players in the Canadian Hockey Association [1]. In the United States, more than 18,000 teams and 200,000 children are currently registered with

USA Hockey [2–4]. In Finland, there are 60,000 registered ice hockey players in a population of five million people, with 45,000 under 19 years of age [5]. Ice hockey is a skilled team sport that has many individual benefits for children and adolescents, including leadership development, team building, discipline, camaraderie, sportsmanship, fun, and cardiovascular conditioning. On the other hand, it is a contact/collision sport that has several inherent features that predispose athletes to injury such as high acceleration and deceleration forces, changing directions, body checking, razor-sharp skates, aggressive stick use, hard rubber projectiles, rigid boards, and a low-friction ice surface. Skating and puck velocities of 32 and 80 km/h, respectively, have been documented for peewee players (age 12 years) [6]. Such characteristics result in frequent high-impact collisions between players, as well as forceful impacts with the side boards, goal posts, pucks, and hockey sticks.

Recently, concern has been expressed, both public and professional, about the increased frequency of injuries in youth leagues that permit body checking, especially as players become bigger, stronger, and faster [1]. At all levels of competition, hockey associations world-wide have tried to reduce the frequency of injuries through rule changes, strict rule enforcement, stiffer penalties for illegal play, enhanced coaching techniques, and the mandation of protective equipment. None of these strategies, however, has been uniformly implemented, primarily because of a lack of scientific evidence to support their effectiveness in reducing injury and philosophical debates among administrators.

This article reviews the distribution and determinants of injuries reported in the pediatric ice hockey literature, and suggests potential injury prevention strategies and directions for further research.

Thirteen electronic databases were searched using a combination of Medical Subject Headings and text words by means of 'wild cards' and Boolean operators to identify potentially relevant English and non-English articles. The search strategy administered was as follows: (1) injur$ OR (athletic injur$) [all fields], AND (2) (child$ OR adolesc$ OR pediatric) [all fields], AND (3) (random$ OR (controlled trial$) OR prospectiv$ OR cohort OR control$ OR compar$ OR (follow-up) OR volunteer$ OR risk OR inciden$ OR rate OR case$ OR cross-section$ OR survey OR questionnaire) [all fields], AND (4) (hockey$ OR (ice hockey$)) [all fields]. The electronic databases and number of citations identified using a combination of the above search strategies are shown in table 1. In addition, the Science Citation Index (1981–2004), Social Sciences Citation Index (1981–2004), and Arts & Humanities Citation Index (1981–2004) data-bases (ISI Web of Science, 1975 to May 2004) were searched by entering a commonly referenced original study [7] pertaining to the topic of interest. Furthermore, 'grey literature' databases and resources were searched, including Dissertations Abstracts (http://www.ucalgary.ca/library/gateway/indabs.html),

Table 1. Electronic search strategy with number of identified citations

Electronic database	Search strategy	Number of citations	Number of potentially relevant citations
MEDLINE (1966–April 2004 week 5)	1 AND 2 AND 3 AND 4	156	48
HealthSTAR (1975–April 2004)	1 AND 2 AND 3 AND 4	126	45
SportDiscuss (1830–1997), (1998–Oct 2003)	1 AND 2 AND 4	108	22
EMBASE (1980–2004 week 20)	1 AND 2 AND 3 AND 4	82	32
PubMed (1966–March 2004)	1 AND 2 AND 3 AND 4	181	45
CINAHL (1982–May 2004 week 1)	1 AND 2 AND 3 AND 4	125	14
OLDMEDLINE (1951–1965)	1 AND 2 AND 3 AND 4	0	0
Biological Abstracts (1980–March 2004)	1 AND 2 AND 3 AND 4	26	15
AMED – Allied and Complementary Medicine (1985–May 2004)	1 AND 2 AND 3 AND 4	1	1
Cochrane Database of Systematic Reviews (1st Quarter 2004)	1 AND 2 AND 4	3	0
ACP Journal Club (1991 to Jan/Feb 2004)	1 AND 2 AND 3 AND 4	0	0
Database of Abstracts of Reviews of Effects (1st Quarter 2004)	1 AND 2 AND 4	0	0
Cochrane Central Register of Controlled Trials (1st Quarter 2004)	1 AND 2 AND 4	0	0

Health Canada (http://www.hc-sc.gc.ca/english/ index.htm), and general internet searching via Google. Lastly, the bibliographies of the selected articles were hand-searched to identify additional articles not identified using the above search strategies.

Selection Criteria

The following predetermined inclusion criteria were used to select relevant studies: (1) original data (cross-sectional, case series, case control, prospective cohort, quasi-experimental, and randomized controlled trials); (2) injuries sustained in the sport of ice hockey; (3) injuries sustained by children 18 years or younger; (4) male or female athletes; (5) athletes participating at all levels of competition; (6) peer-reviewed reports/articles; and (7) English language. Exclusion criteria were as follows: (1) studied injuries related to congenital anomalies; (2) studied injury rates among a broad age spectrum of athletes, including pediatric and adult hockey players; (3) review articles, commentaries, case reports, letters to the editor, and anecdotal reports; (4) studied specific injuries over a broad range of sport settings (i.e., study not exclusive to the sport of ice hockey); and (5) non-English articles. Because there was a scarcity of peer-reviewed studies pertaining to ice hockey injuries on children 18 years of age and younger, we included studies reporting injuries among athletes participating at the Junior level of competition (ages 15–20 years).

The titles and abstracts (when available) of the identified citations were screened by one investigator to identify all potentially relevant articles. If insufficient information was available (e.g., no abstract), the full papers were reviewed for inclusion based on the predetermined selection criteria. A comparison between studies on this topic area was difficult because of the following limitations:

- The majority of studies were observational descriptive, with very few analytical designs.
- The definition of the outcome variable (i.e., injury) was not clearly stated in several of the selected studies. For example, an overestimation of injury rates may occur if all injuries were reported, regardless of the reporting source (e.g., coach, parent). In addition, questionnaires with no clearly stated injury definition may underestimate injury rates if athletes were required to self-report injuries retrospectively, especially if no time loss from participation was experienced. Furthermore, concussion rates would be significantly underestimated if they were defined as 'any loss of consciousness experienced by a player during contact, whether a momentary loss of consciousness or an amnesia-type disorder' because greater than 90% of sport-related concussions do not result in loss of consciousness [8].
- Data collection methods ranged from self-report to insurance claim, coach, therapist, and physician report.
- The validity of the recording mechanisms was unknown in the majority of studies pertaining to the topic of interest.
- The study populations were generally small, with no reported sample size or power calculations.
- There was no standardization of injury incidence (e.g., injuries per 1,000 athlete-exposures or 1,000 player-hours) in several studies, and individual participation (exposure) information was rarely collected; this is critical for the assessment of risk.

- Study populations were predominantly samples of convenience with no random selection of subjects, a source of selection bias.
- Individual baseline injury history was not reported in several studies; this may have resulted in an overestimation of injury rates if the athletes selected were more likely to be injured based on their previous injury history (that is, if there was differential participation).
- There was no report of subject drop-outs or loss to follow-up in several of the selected studies; this may have lead to an underestimation of association between specific risk factors and injury (if the reason for drop-out was related to the injury itself).
- A significant source of bias in the reviewed studies was a lack of measurement and control for potentially confounding variables. Differences in coaching techniques, musculature and cardiovascular conditioning, warm-up routines, protective equipment use, rules, rule enforcement, age, experience level, skill level, position, previous injury history, venue type (i.e., practice vs. game), and arena characteristics may all have a significant effect on the results.
- External validity of the results in several of the selected studies was limited due to the lack of internal validity.

Incidence of Injury

Incidence is defined by Last [9] as 'the number of new events, e.g., new cases of a disease [or injury in this case] in a defined population, within a specified period of time'. Incidence rate is 'the rate at which new events occur in a population. The numerator is the number of new events that occur in a defined population; the denominator is the population at risk of experiencing the event during this period, sometimes expressed as person-time' [9].

Table 2 highlights a comparison of injury rates among ice hockey players participating at the Junior level of play and under [2, 3, 5, 7, 10–29]. As shown in the table, there was a wide range of injury rates reported in the studies selected for review. It was impossible to give a single approximation or range for the rate of ice hockey injuries sustained. This can be attributed to differences in study design (prospective vs. retrospective), differences between the sample population at risk of injury (e.g., associations, leagues, age groups, levels of play, equipment rules, and officiating rules), different sources of injury collection (e.g., players, coaches, trainers, therapists, physicians, emergency department visits, insurance claims, databases), different methods for measuring athlete participation (exposure) time (e.g., estimation vs. direct observation; player-hours, athlete-exposures), different methods of calculating

Table 2. A comparison of injury rates among pediatric ice hockey players

Level/Study	Design P/R	Injury collection (source)	Age (years)	Duration of study(number of seasons and year)	Sample number of subjects	Sample number of teams	Number of injuries	Injury rate			
								injuries per game	injuries per 100 players	injuries per 1,000 h	injuries per 1,000 A-E
Junior											
[2]	P	Trainer and MD	17–20	3 (1990–1993)	25	1	142			9.4	
[10]	P	MD and trainers	16–20 (?)	1	22	1	74		Fwd: 138	Games Def: 151	
[21]	P / R	Trainers, coaches, MDs	15–20	2 (1998–2000)	Year 1: 272 Year 2: 283	14	Year 1: 29 Year 2: 21		Year 1: 10.7 Year 2: 7.42	Games Year 1: 5.95 Year 2: 4.63	
[13]	P	?	15–19	1 (1977–1978)	?	1	83				
[22]	P	Trainers	16–21	1 ?	282	10	Head, neck, face only 113			NFS: 158.9 HS: 73.5 FS: 23.2	
[16]	R	Trainer and athletic therapists	16–20	1 (1993–1994)	?	16	328	LTS: 0.33 S: 0.58 STS: 0.76			
High School											
[7]	R	Quest.	Mean 16.1	1 (1982–1983)	251	12	75 per 100 players		75	5	
[17]	P	Athletic trainers	<20	1 (1994)	273	16	29			Total: 135.6 FP: 89.7 RR: 294.1	Total: 26.4 FP: 17 RR: 64.5
[23]	P	MDs	JV: 15–18 V: 16–19	1 (1994–1995)	JV: 39 V: 47	JV: 3 V: 3	JV: 10 V: 17			JV: 30.3 V: 49.7	
[24]	R	Quest.	14–18	2 (1982–1984)	480	12	Shoulder only 45		9.4		
[25]	P	Coaches/ trainers	?	1 (1974–1975)	207	11	41			62.1	

Table 2. (continued)

Level/Study	Design P/R	Injury collection (source)	Age (years)	Duration of study (number of seasons and year)	Sample number of subjects	Sample number of teams	Number of injuries	Injury rate			
								injuries per game	injuries per 100 players	injuries per 1,000 h	injuries per 1,000 A-E
Minor											
[26]	R	Insurance and Federal Stats	14–20	1987–1989	29,911	?	1,570			86	
[20]	P	Emerg./ Quest.	7–18	1995–1996	103	n/a	113				
[15]	P	Managers/ coaches	9–15	1 (1990–1991)	150	9	52		35		
[12]	P	Quest.	9–18	1 (1990–1991)	1,437	54	128		<12 years: 0.88 12–15 years: 12.4 15–18 years: 25.3		
[3]	P	MD	9–14	1 (1993–1994)	66	4	14			9–10 years: 1.0 11–12 years: 1.8 13–14 years: 4.3	
[14]	P	Survey	12–13	1 (1985–1986)	279	BC (AA): 6 BC (CC): 22 NBC (CC): 21	BC (AA): 19 BC (CC): 26 NBC (CC): 7				
[19]	P	Survey	14–15	2 (1987–1989)	?	Minor: 37 Major: 44	Minor: 632 Major: 132	Minor: 2.08 Major: 0.12			
[11]	R	Patient records	6–15	3 (1980–1982)	1,124 sport-related injuries	N/A (emergency patients)	290 (26%)				

Ref		Data source	Age	Years (period)	Exposures		Injuries		Injury rate
[27]	P	Self-report and CHA	Atom	3 (1998–2001)	Year 1: ODMHA 1,035, OHF 1,110 Year 2: ODMHA 885, OHF 1,515 Year 3: ODMHA 4,232, OHF 53,920	Year 1: 143 Year 2: 160 Year 3: 136	Year 1: ODMHA 12, OHF 6 Year 2: ODMHA 16, OHF 25 Year 3: ODMHA 63, OHF 273		Year 1: ODMHA 1.16, OHF 0.54 Year 2: ODMHA 1.81, OHF 1.65 Year 3: ODMHA 1.49, OHF 0.80
[28]	P	Athletic trainer	11–19	1 (1993–1994)	807	?	Boys: 60 Girls: 4		Boys: 117.3 Girls: 50.5
[18]	R	Quest./survey	12–13	1 (1985–1986)	279	BC (AA): 6 BC (CC): 22 NBC (CC): 21	BC (CC): 54 NBC (CC): 16	BC (CC): 2.84 NBC (CC): 0.67	
[5]	R	Insurance company	≤11 12–14 15–19	1 (1996)	15,706 15,363 11,157	?	Upper extremity only 20 126 304		injuries per 1,000 player-years 1.5 9.4 27.2
[29]	P	Interview	Mean: 14.7 SD: 1.6	1 (1997–1998)	78 females	?	32		41
[25]	P	Coaches/trainers	5–14	1 (1974–1975)	706	40	17	10	6.7

LTS = Larger than standard ice surface (>17,000 ft²); S = standard ice surface (200 × 85 ft – 17,000 ft²); STS = < standard ice surface (<17,000 ft²); SD = standard deviation.

Minor = An injury as the result of a blow that damages the integrity of human tissue and causes a temporary incapacity (a shift missed) on the part of the player injured.

Major = An injury as the result of a blow that damages the integrity of human tissue creating a state of incapacity that prevents the person from playing or practicing during a certain period of time.

A-E = athlete-exposures; P = prospective; R = retrospective; V = varsity; JV = junior varsity; NFS = no face shield; HS = half shield; FS = full shield; FP = fair play rules; RR = regular rules; BC (AA) = body checking, level AA; BC (CC) = body checking, level CC; NBC (CC) = no body checking, level CC.

injury rates (e.g., incidence: injuries per 1,000 athlete-exposures, injuries per 1,000 player-hours, prevalence: injuries per 100 players), and varying definitions of injury (time loss vs. no time loss vs. specific anatomical injuries). Retrospective studies identified injury prevalence within a specific team or league and were less accurate in identifying the true population at risk of injury.

Injury Characteristics

Injury Location
The reported hockey-related anatomic injury locations across the entire body are shown in Table 3 [2, 3, 5, 7, 10–13, 15, 17, 18, 22, 23, 25, 28, 29]. Players competing at the Minor hockey level sustained most of their injuries to the upper extremity (23–55%; shoulder, 11.6–22%; arm, 3.9–23%), followed by the spine/trunk (13–32.8%; chest/ribs, 7.7–14%; neck, 7–9.7%; back, 7–9.6%), head (7–30%), and lower extremity (21–27%; knee, 7–9.6%; leg, 3.9–27%; thigh, 3.9–7%). At the High School level, the head was the primary anatomic area injured, accounting for between 14.8% and 31% of the total injuries sustained. The lower extremity was the next most common injured part of the body (20.6–37%; knee, 6.9–14.8%; thigh, 6.9–11.1%), followed by the upper extremity (3.4–29%; shoulder, 3.4–16%;), and spine/trunk (7.4–17.2%; chest/ribs, 6.9–7.4%; back, 5–6.9%). At the Junior level of competition, the lower extremity was the primary region injured (24.9–33.7%; pelvis/hips, 4.2–14%; knee, 4.2–13.3%; thigh, 4–12.8%), followed by the upper extremity (9.6–35.4%; shoulder, 4.8–20%; hand/fingers, 5–16.7%), the head (14.4–28%; face, 9.6–29.2%), and the spine/trunk (6–14.9%; neck, 1–8.5%; back, 2.1–8.3%).

There was a dramatic decrease in the proportion of head and neck injury insurance claims by 8–16-year-old United States amateur hockey players from 45% during the 1975–1976 season to 36% the season after the American Society of Testing Materials standard, 'Eye and Face Protective Equipment for Hockey Players' (F513–77), was passed [30]. The American Society of Testing Materials is a voluntary organization which develops consensus standards for thousands of materials, systems, and products which are used in society – a subcommittee representing ice hockey was asked by the Amateur Hockey Association of the United States to develop a standard for facial protection [30]. Claims dropped to 31% during the 1977–1978 season and remained at that level through to the 1983–1984 season. In addition, dental claims dropped greater than 50% from 1975 to 1984 [30]. Kvist et al. [11] studied sport-related injury profiles of children aged 6–15 years treated in the Turku University Central Hospital Casualty Department from 1980 to 1982. Twenty-six percent (290/1,124) of the

Table 3. A percent comparison of injury location among pediatric ice hockey players

Injuries	Junior (%)				High School (%)					Minor (%)							
	[2]	[13]	[10]	[22]	[7]	[17]	[25]	[23]	[28]	[15]	[12]	[3]	[11]	[18]	[5]	[29]	[25]
Total no. injuries	142	83	74	(head, neck, facial only) 113	75/100 players	29	41	27	Boys: 60 Girls: 4	52	128	14	290	BC (CC): 54 NBC (CC): 16	(upper extremity only) ≤11:20 12–14: 126 15–19: 304	32 (females only)	17
Head	2				19			68.2	14.8	9.6	10		7	BC (CC): 16.7 NBC (CC): 12.5		6.3 (including neck)	58.7
Face	26	9.6	Fwd: 23.4, Def: 29.2	58		6.9			Head and neck	3.9							
Teeth		4.8	1.4	14		0											
Concussion			0	13		13.8			Boys: 30 Girls: 0	2.3			10				
Eye		0	0	12		15.8	2.4			0	13						
Spine/Trunk								7.4						BC (CC): 24.1 NBC (CC): 31.3		31.3	5.9
Neck	1		Fwd: 8.5, Def: 4.2	0.9	3	3.4				9.7	7	7	7	BC (CC): 16.7 NBC (CC): 6.25			
Upper back	4.8		Back		Back	Back	Back			Back							
Lower back	6		Fwc: 2.1, Def: 8.3		5	6.9	4.9			9.6							
Chest/Ribs	2		Fwd: 4.3, Def: 0		7	6.9		7.4		7.7		14					
Abdomen	1	0	0		2	0				5.8							
Upper extremity											55						
Shoulder	20	4.8	Fwd: 12.8, Def: 12.5		16	3.4	2.4	11.1	11.6	11.6		22	22	BC (CC): 16.7 NBC (CC): 12.5	≤11: 0.5 12–14: 11 15–19: 35	21.9	5.9
Arm			Fwd: 2.1, Def: 0		13	0			Boys: 23 Girls: 0	3.9							

Table 3 (continued)

Injuries	Junior (%)				High School (%)				Minor (%)								
	[2]	[13]	[10]	[22]	[7]	[17]	[25]	[23]	[28]	[15]	[12]	[3]	[11]	[18]	[5]	[29]	[25]
Total no. injuries	142	83	74	(head, neck, facial only) 113	75/100 players	29	41	27	Boys: 60 Girls: 4	52	128	14	290	BC (CC): 54 NBC (CC): 16	(upper extremity only) ≤11:20 12–14: 126 15–19: 304	32 (females only)	17
Hand/Fingers	5		Fwd: 6.4, Def: 16.7			0		7.4		7.7							
Elbow	2	4.8	Fwd: 6.4, Def: 0			0				5.8					≤11: 3 12–14: 16 15–19: 48		
Forearm			Fwd: 2.1, Def: 2.0			0				0							
Wrist	1		Fwd: 0, Def: 4.2			0		3.7		1.9							
Lower extremity											19			BC (CC): 24.1 NBC (CC): 37.5		40.6	
Pelvis/Hips	14		Fwd: 6.4, Def: 4.2		4		4.9	11.1		1.9							
Thigh	4	6.0	Fwd: 12.8, Def: 12.5			6.9	4.9	11.1		3.9		7					5.9
Knee	6	13.3	Fwd: 8.5, Def: 4.2		10	6.9	4.9	14.8		9.6		7					23.5
Leg	1	1.2	Fwd: 2.1, Def: 0		11	0	2.4		Boys: 27 Girls: 50	3.9							
Foot/Toes	5	1.2	Fwd: 2.1, Def: 0			3.4				0		7					
Ankle	4	3.6	Fwd: 0, Def: 4.2		5	3.4				3.8							

BC (CC) = Body checking, level CC; NBC (CC) = no body checking, level CC.
Note: If cell is blank, either no injury occurred or data was not reported.

total reported sport-related injuries were sustained in ice hockey (boys: 24.9%; girls: 1%). Thirty-four percent of the hockey-related injuries were to the head and neck, and approximately two-thirds (65%) of the total dental injuries and 3.7% of fractures sustained by boys occurred in ice hockey. Bjorkenheim et al. [12] studied the risk and type of injuries sustained by 1437 players (aged 9–18 years) who were required to wear full facial protection in an organized junior league in Helsinki. Only 1% of the 682 ice hockey players aged 9–12 years were injured, compared with 14% of the 534 players aged 12–15, and 23% of the 221 players aged 15–18 years [12]. These results suggest that teenagers were the most vulnerable to hockey-related injuries caused by direct trauma. Of note, 32% of the total injuries were caused by an illegal play. Park and Castaldi [13] studied the types and frequency of game injuries sustained by players aged 15–19 years from one Junior 'B' hockey team during the 1977–1978 season. Facial injuries were the most frequent type (22.6%), followed by knee injuries (13.3%), hip and forearm/arm injuries (7.2% each), and thigh and groin injuries (6.0% each), respectively. Pinto et al. [10] studied injuries sustained by 16–20-year-old players from one Junior 'A' hockey team over the course of one season. The most common site of injury was the face, accounting for 24.3% of the total injuries. The shoulder and hand/fingers were the next most common injured area (12.2% each), followed by the knee and thigh (9.5% each).

Situational

Table 4 highlights injury rates reported during practices and games for the studies selected for review [2, 3, 7, 10, 12, 15, 20, 21, 23, 24, 29]. An overwhelming majority of injuries were sustained during games compared with practices. Pinto et al. [10] studied injuries sustained by 16–20-year-old players from one Junior 'A' hockey team over the course of a season. The injury rate during games was more than 20 times the rate during practices, and exhibition and preseason games had an injury rate greater than 3 times that of regular season and postseason games. Stuart and Smith [2] studied the incidence and types of injuries sustained during practices and games for one US Junior 'A' hockey team over 3 consecutive seasons. Players were 25 times more likely to be injured during games than practices. Overall, the percent of total injuries sustained during games ranged from 58 to 96.3, with a rate between 4.63 injuries per 1,000 hours and 143 injuries per 1,000 hours. In practices, injury rates ranged from zero to 23 injuries per 1,000 hours, with injuries accounting for between 3.7 and 37% of the total reported injuries.

Action or Activity

Table 5 shows the mechanism of injury for the studies selected for review [2, 3, 5, 7, 10, 12–14, 15–25, 28, 29, 31–33]. In Junior hockey, the primary

Table 4. A comparison of injury rates in practices versus games among pediatric ice hockey players

Level/ Study	Design P/R	Number of subjects	Number of injuries	Duration of study (seasons)	Practice		Game	
					percent of total number of injuries	injuries per 1,000h	percent of total number of injuries	injuries per 1,000h
Junior								
[2]	P	25	142	3	37	3.9	58	96.1
[10]	P	22	74	1	23	4	62	Exhibition: 303 League/ postseason: 83
[21]	P and R	Year 1: 272 Year 2: 283	Year 1: 29 Year 2: 21	2		Year 1: 0.6 Year 2: 0		Year 1: 5.95 Year 2: 4.63
High School								
[7]	R	251	?	1			82.3	
[23]	P	86	27	1	3.7		96.3	Junior varsity: 30.3 Varsity: 49.7
[24]	R	480	Shoulder only 45	2	25		63	
Minor Hockey								
[20]	P	103	113	1	17		83	
[15]	P	150	52	1	15	23	85	143
[12]	P	1,437	128	1	6		94	
[3]	P	66	9–10 years: 1 11–12 years: 2 13–14 years: 11	1		1.1 2.2 2.5		0 0 10.9
[29]	P	78 females	32	1	7		93	

P = Prospective; R = retrospective.

Table 5. A percent comparison of mechanism of injury among pediatric ice hockey players

Level/ Study	Age (years)	Sample number of subjects	Sample number of teams	Duration (number of seasons and year)	Number of injuries	Illegal play (%)	Body check/ collision (%)	Stick contact (%)	Puck contact (%)	Skate contact (%)	Fall (%)	Other (%)
Junior												
[2]	17–20	25	1	3 (1990–1993)	142		24	14	11	3		48
[10]	16–20	22	1	1 ?	74	20	12.2	16.2			12.2	
[21]	15–20	Year 1: 272 Year 2: 283	14	2 (1998–2000)	Year 1: 29 Year 2: 21	Year 1: ? Year 2: 35.8		Year 1: 7 Year 2: 4	Year 1: 6 Year 2: 3			
[13]	15–19	?	1	1 (1977–1978)	83		48	12	17		7	16
[16]	16–20	?	16	1 (1993–1994)	328	Penalties/ game LTS: 20.2 S: 19.0 STS: 18.8						
[22]	16–21	282	10	1 ?	113 (head, neck, facial only)	16.5	28.3	36.3	6.2		6.2	23
High School												
[7]	Mean 16.1	251	12	1 (1982–1983)	75 per 100 players		74.4		7.5		8	
[17]	<20	273	16	1 (1994)	29	21.4	67.9	14.3	14.3	3.6	0	0
[23]	15–19	86	6	1 (1994–1995)	27		74.1	11.1	0	3.7		11.1
[24]	14–18	480	12	2 (1982–1984)	Shoulder only 45	43	24.4	6.8	2.2			66.6
[25]	?	207	11	1 (1974–1975)	41	29.1						

Ice Hockey

Table 5 (continued)

Level/ Study	Age (years)	Sample number of subjects	Sample number of teams	Duration (number of seasons and year)	Number of injuries	Illegal play (%)	Body check/ collision (%)	Stick contact (%)	Puck contact (%)	Skate contact (%)	Fall (%)	Other (%)
Minor												
[20]	7–18	103	n/a	1 (1995–1996)	113	26.3	57	7.8	7.8	2.9	5.8	1.9
[15]	9–15	150	9	1 (1990–1991)	52	66	86					
[12]	9–18	1,437	54	1 (1990–1991)	128	32	44.5	22.7	25			7.8
[3]	9–14	66	4	1 (1993–1994)	14		50	7.1	14.3	7.1	7.1	14.3
[19]	14–15	?	37	2 (1987–1989)	Minor: 632 Major: 132		Minor: 51.4 Major: 76.5	Minor: 25.8 Major: 6.4	Minor: 13.1 Major: 2.3		Minor: 6.3 Major: 7.4	Minor: 3.4 Major: 6.85
[14]	12–13	279	BC (A): 6 BC (C): 22 NBC (C): 21	1 (1985–1986)	Fractures BC (A): 11 BC (C): 14 NBC (C): 1	Regular season BC: 12.4/ game NBC: 9.1/ game Tournament BC: 8.2/ game NBC: 6.8/ game	Fractures BC (A): 91 BC (C): 86 NBC (C): 0				Fractures BC (A): 0 BC (C): 0 NBC (C): 100	
[28]	11–19	807	?	1 (1993–1994)	Boys: 60 Girls: 4 Eye only		Boys: 65 Girls: 50	Boys: 17 Girls: 25	Boys: 13 Girls: 25	Boys: 2 Girls: 0		Boys: 2 Girls: 0

[31]	≤10 11–15 16–20	?	?	1 (1974–1975)	28 76 56	62	31				7
[32]	<11 11–15 16–20	?	?	1 (1976–1977)	Eye only 10 18 25	56	36				6.7
[33]	≤10 11–15 16–20	?	?	1 (1983–1984)	Eye only 6 18 22	52	44				4
[18]	12–13	279	BC (A): 6 BC (C): 22 NBC (C): 21	1 (1985–1986)	BC (C): 54 NBC (C): 16	BC (C): 55.5 NBC (C): 18.8 (opponent contact)	BC (C): 22.2 NBC (C): 18.8	BC (C): 5.6 NBC (C): 18.8	BC (C): 1.9 NBC (C): 0	BC (C): 5.6 NBC (C): 12.5	BC (C): 9.4 NBC (C): 31.3
[5]	≤11 12–14 15–19	13,706 13,363 11,157	?	1 (1996)	? 126 304 Upper extremity only 20	30 53.2 54.6	10 6.3 8.9	15 7.9 10.2	0	35 17.5 13.2	10 15.1 13.2
[29]	Mean: 14.7	78 females	?	1 (1997–98)	32	56.3	25	9.4	0	3.1	6.2

LTS = Larger than standard ice surface (>17,000 ft²); S = standard ice surface (200 × 85 ft = 17,000 ft²); STS = smaller than standard ice surface (<17,000 ft²). BC (A) = Body checking, level AA; BC (C) = body checking, level CC; NBC (C) = no body checking, level CC.
Note: If cell is blank, specific mechanism was not reported.

mechanism of injury was body checking (12.2–48%), followed by puck contact (3–17%), and stick contact (4–16.2%). Illegal play reportedly caused between 16.5 and 35.8% of the total injuries at this level of competition. In High School hockey, body checking was again the most common cause of injury ranging from 67.9–74.1% of the total reported injuries. Stick contact was the second most common (11.1–14.3%), followed by puck contact (0–14.3%). Illegal play reportedly caused between 21.4 and 29.1% of the injuries. Similarly, body checking was the predominant mechanism of injury at the Minor hockey level (50–86%), followed by stick contact (6.4–25.8%), and puck contact (2.3–14.3%). Illegal play was involved in 26.3–66% of injuries.

Injury Severity

Injury Types

Table 6 shows a percent comparison of the different types of injuries sustained by pediatric ice hockey players, separated by level of competition [2, 3, 5, 7, 10–15, 17–20, 22–25, 28, 29]. In Junior hockey, the three most common reported types of injuries were sprains/strains (20.5–41%), contusions (18–45.8%), and lacerations (9.6–24%). Similarly, the most frequent types of injuries in High School hockey were contusions (29–58.6%), sprains/strains (6.8–37%), lacerations (10.3–13%), and concussions (3.7–13.8%). The most common injury types sustained in Minor hockey were contusions (13–64.9%), sprains/strains (10–32.2%), fractures (2.4–54%), concussions (5–43%), and lacerations (5.6–19%). Regnier et al. [14] showed that the rate of fractures was 12 times greater for Pee-Wee level players competing in a league that allowed body checking compared with one that did not allow any body checking.

Catastrophic Injury

Table 7 highlights catastrophic injury rates among pediatric ice hockey players [30–34]. Catastrophic injuries were defined as those injuries that caused death or permanent disability. In 1973, a Canadian ophthalmologist, Dr. Tom Pashby, investigated ocular injuries among Canadian amateur hockey players and reported that 287 hockey-related eye injuries were treated by members of the Canadian Ophthalmologic Society during one season, 20 of which resulted in blindness [31]. Similarly, during the 1974–1975 Canadian amateur season, 257 ocular injuries were treated with 43 instances of legal blindness [32]. In the United States, the Consumer Products Safety Commission reported an increase in amateur ice hockey injuries from 30,000 to 50,000 between 1973 and 1975, two-thirds of which involved the head/face and 5–9% the eye [35]. Results

Table 6. A percent comparison of injury types among pediatric ice hockey players

Level/Study	Age (years)	Total number of injuries	Dental (%)	Concussion (%)	Fracture (%)	Laceration (%)	Contusion (%)	Sprain (%)	Strain (%)	Dislocation (%)	Other (%)
Junior											
[2]	17–20	142	4		4	24	18	16	25		
[10]	16–20	74	?	Fwd: 2.1 Def: 0	Fwd: 8.5 Def: 4.2	Fwd: 14.9 Def: 20.8	Fwd: 29.8 Def: 29.2	Fwd: 36.2 Def: 41.7			Fwd: 8.5 Def: 4.2
[13]	15–19	83	4.7		2.4	9.6	45.8	10.9	9.6		
[22]	16–21	113 (head, neck, facial only)	6.2	9	4.4	70	3.5	1.8			Eye: 1
High School											
[7]	Mean 16.1	75/100 players		12	11	13	29	14		3	14
[17]	<20	29	0	13.8	6.9	10.3	58.6	3.4	3.4	0	0
[23]	15–19	27	0	3.7	7.4	11.1	37	22.2	14.8	3.7	
[24]	14–18	Shoulder only 45	n/a	n/a	4.4	2.2	17.9	42.2	22.2	subluxations	4.4
[25]	?	41		7.3						6.8	
Minor Hockey											
[28]	11–19	Boys: 60 Girls: 4	Boys: 0 Girls: 0	Boys: 15 Girls: 0		Boys: 6.5 Girls: 0	Boys: 60 Girls: 100	Boys: 10 Girls: 0			Boys: 8.5 Girls: 0
[20]	7–18	113		16	20	19	13	6	5	1	20
[15]	9–15	52		9	8	2	50	6	13	4	8
[12]	9–18	128	2.3		25						
[3]	9–14	14	0	0	29	7	36	21		0	7

Table 6 (continued)

Level/Study	Age (years)	Total number of injuries	Dental (%)	Concussion (%)	Fracture (%)	Laceration (%)	Contusion (%)	Sprain (%)	Strain (%)	Dislocation (%)	Other (%)
[14]	12–13	BC (AA): 19 BC (CC): 26 NBC (CC): 7		BC (AA): 5 BC (CC): 15 NBC (CC): 43	BC (AA): 58 BC (CC): 54 NBC (CC): 14			BC (AA): 21 BC (CC): 23 NBC (CC): 29		BC (AA): 16 BC (CC): 8 NBC (CC): 14	
[11]	6–15	290	10		Boys: 2.4						
[19]	14–15	Minor: 632 Major: 132		Minor: ? Major: 15.6	Minor: ? Major: 28.6	Minor: 5.6 Major: ?	Minor: 64.9 Major: ?	Minor: ? Major: 32.2		Minor: ? Major: 8.6	Minor: 29.7 Major: 14.1
[18]	12–13	BC (CC): 54 NBC (CC): 16		BC (CC): 1.9 NBC (CC): 6.3	BC: n = 25 NBC: n = 1	BC (CC): 1.9 NBC (CC): 0	BC (CC): 72.2 NBC (CC): 68.8		BC (CC): 3.7 NBC (CC): 6.3	BC: n = 5 NBC: n = 1	BC (CC): 20.4 NBC (CC): 18.8
[5]	≤11 12–14 15–19	Upper extremity 20 126 304			4 22 44						
[29]	Mean: 14.7	32 (females only)	0	3.1	3.1	0	50	37.5		0	6.3
[25]	5–14	17		11.7							

BC (AA) = Body checking, level AA; BC (CC) = body checking, level CC; NBC (CC) = no body checking, level CC.

Minor = An injury as the result of a blow that damages the integrity of human tissue and causes a temporary incapacity (a shift missed) on the part of the player injured.

Major = An injury as the result of a blow that damages the integrity of human tissue creating a state of incapacity that prevents the person from playing or practicing during a certain period of time.

Note: If cell is blank, either no injury occurred or data was not reported.

Table 7. A comparison of catastrophic injury rates among pediatric ice hockey players

Study	Number of subjects	Age (years)	Duration (years)	Injury type	Condition	Absolute number	Rate Number per 1,000 athletes
[30]	~700,000	5–14	1973–1980	?	Death		0.0029
[34]	147/241	11–20	Case-series	Cervical spine injury	Fatality	8/241	
					Permanent injury	108/207	
			1966–1993		Complete cord injury	52/207	
[31]	?	≤10	1974–1975	Eye injury	(blind)	28, blind: 5	
		11–15				76, blind: 6	
		16–20				56, blind: 9	
[32]	?	<11	1976–1977	Eye injury	(blind)	10, blind: 0	
		11–15				18, blind: 1	
		16–20				29, blind: 5	
[33]	?	≤10	1983–1984	Eye injury	(blind)	6, blind: 0	
		11–15				18, blind: 0	
		16–20				22, blind: 0	

from studies such as these were instrumental in encouraging hockey administrators to implement mandatory full face shield rules in 1976 for all United States players under the age of 20, and in 1977–1978 for all United States College players [36]. The Canadian Amateur Hockey Association followed this initiative and mandated full facial protection in 1978 for all athletes under its jurisdiction [36].

Research conducted after the implementation of these rules showed a marked reduction in facial and ocular injuries [33, 37–39]. For example, although 93 eye injuries were treated by members of the Canadian Ophthalmologic Society during the 1986–1987 season (compared with 257 in 1974–1975), with 18 instances of legal blindness (compared with 43 in 1974–1975), no eye injuries were sustained by players wearing Canadian Standard Association approved face shields [38]. Several of the studies reviewed in this chapter have shown that the use of protective face shields has been associated with a dramatic decrease in the incidence of eye, facial, and dental injuries. Reynen and Clancy [36] reported that the United States has prevented approximately 420,000 eye injuries and saved roughly $60 million in medical expenses from 1982–1988 as a result of enforcing these rules. Despite such policy changes, head injuries remain a major area for concern across many different age groups and levels of play. Brust et al. [15] ascertained that head injuries accounted for 13.6% of the total reported injuries sustained by children 9–15 years from 9 community teams in Minnesota during the 1990–1991 season. Gerberich et al. [7] studied injury rates among 263 hockey players from 12 US high schools during the 1982–1983 seasons and found that 22% of the total reported injuries were to the head and neck. Kelly et al. [40] retrospectively reviewed medical records from five emergency departments in Edmonton, Alberta to examine the epidemiology of sport-related head injuries (skull fracture, loss of consciousness, or concussion) presenting to the emergency department in 1996–1997; patients <20 years old were involved in 66% of all head injury cases, with 21% occurring in ice hockey [40].

Although mandatory full face shield rules do reduce the frequency of facial and eye injuries in this sport, an alarming increase in hockey-related cervical spine injuries became apparent soon after the initiation of these policy changes. Subsequently, a Committee on Prevention of Spinal Cord Injuries Due to Hockey was formed in 1981 to rigorously investigate this area. Since its formation, the committee has been distributing surveys/questionnaires every 2 years to Canadian neurosurgeons, orthopedic surgeons, physiatrists, and recently sport medicine physicians to document the frequency of major spinal cord injuries occurring in Canadian hockey. By 1993, 241 fractures and dislocations of the spine were entered into the registry, with or without injury to the spinal cord or nerve roots [34]. The registry also showed that the annual incidence of major spinal injuries, excluding all minor injuries to the neck such as sprains and strains, had markedly increased since 1981, averaging 16.8 cases per year from 1982 to 1993 [34]. More alarming, greater than 50% of the spinal cord injuries involved permanent damage, and 25% of the injured players were paralyzed below the level of the injury. Of the 212 cases with adequate documentation, 17.5% of the athletes were 11–15 years of age, and 51.9% were between 16 and 20 years [34]. The main mechanism of hockey-related cervical spine injuries was an axial load on the head with a flexed neck during a collision with the boards, goal posts, or another player, forcing the cervical spine into compression [34, 41–45]. The most common site of injury was the C5-C6 region, and burst fractures and fracture-dislocations were the most frequent types of vertebral injuries [34]. In addition, Molsa et al. [46] studied the incidence and mechanisms of ice hockey-related major spinal cord injury in Finland and Sweden from 1980–1996. Six of the sixteen cases involving permanent neurological deficits (37.5%) were ice hockey players aged 14–19 years [46].

Time Loss

Table 8 highlights a comparison of injury severity between several of the selected studies, as measured by time loss from competition, hospitalization, and fractures [2, 3, 5, 7, 11, 14, 15, 17, 24, 28, 29]. Few studies addressed

Table 8. A comparison of injury severity among pediatric ice hockey players

Study	Design P/R	Age(s)	Year	Number of injuries	Time loss	Hospitalization
[11]	R	6–15	1980–1982	290/1,124		23/290
[28]	P	11–19	1993–1994	Boys: 60 Girls: 4	Boys: >7 d 18% Girls: >7 d 0%	
[2]	P	17–20	1990–1993	142	*Mild: 58% Moderate: 36% Severe: 6%	Surgery:2.1%
[7]	R	Mean: 16.1	1982–1983	75 per 100 players	**Mild: 54% Moderate: 28% Severe: 18%	
[15]	P	9–15	1990–1991	52	‡Minimal: 56% Minor: 27% Moderate: 11% Major: 6%	
[3]	P	9–14	1993–1994	14	†Mild: 57% Moderate: 7% Severe: 36%	
[14]	P	12–13	1985–1996	Fractures BC (A): 1 per 8.2 games BC (C): 1 per 22.5 games NBC (C): 1 per 263 games		
[17]	P	<20	1994	29	≤1 day: 60.7% >1 day, FL, or C: 39.3%	

Table 8 (continued)

Study	Design	Age(s)	Year	Number of injuries	Time loss
[28]	P	11–19	1993–1994	Boys: 60 Girls: 4	Boys: ≤1 day: 57% Boys: >7 days: 18%
[5]	R	≤11 12–14 15–19	1996	Upper extremity only 20 126 304	≤11 †Minor: 1% / Moderate: 5% / Major: 1% 12–14 Minor: 15% / Moderate: 13% / Major: 20% 15–19 Minor: 36% / Moderate: 39% / Major: 43%
[24]	R	14–18	1982–1984	Shoulder only 45	†††Minor: 33.3 Moderate: 37.8 Major: 15.6
[29]	P	Mean: 14.7	1997–1998	32 (females only)	††Minor: 84.4 Moderate: 9.4 Major: 6.3

FL = Facial Laceration, C = concussion, BC (A) = body checking, level AA; NBC (C) = no body checking, level CC; P = prospective; R = retrospective.

*Mild = ≤3 days missed; moderate = 4–14 days missed; severe = long-term sequela expected and athlete unable to return in same capacity.

**Mild = ≤1 week time loss; moderate = 1–3 weeks time loss; severe = >3 weeks time loss.

†Minimal = ≤1 day time loss; minor = 2–7 days time loss; moderate = 8–24 days time loss; major = ≥25 days time loss.

†Mild = ≤3 days missed; moderate = 4–14 days missed; severe = long-term sequela expected and athlete may be unable to return to play in same capacity.

††Minor = ≤7 days missed; moderate = 8–27 days missed; major = ≥28 days missed.

†††Minor = <1 week missed; moderate = 1–3 weeks missed; major = >3 weeks missed.

injury severity due to the retrospective designs, definitions of injury, and failure to collect time loss information. Among the studies which classified various degrees of severity, large time loss discrepancies made comparison of studies difficult. Hockey-related injuries were the most common of all sport injuries leading to hospitalization among children aged 6–15 years treated in the Turku University Central Hospital Casualty Department from 1980 to 1982 (23/102) [11].

Injury Risk Factors

Specific ice hockey-related injury risk factors are poorly delineated and rarely studied in the pediatric ice hockey literature. Size differences between players competing at the Minor hockey level of competition was one potential risk factor for injury. Weight and height differences between the smallest and largest Bantam hockey players were shown to be 53 kg and 55 cm, respectively [15]. Weight differences were statistically significant, and lighter players were more likely to be injured. In addition, a statistically significant increase in injuries was associated with age, with 54% of the injuries sustained by Bantam players (ages 13–15), 27% by Peewee players (ages 11–13), and 19% by Squirts (ages 9–11) [15]. Roy et al. [18] evaluated morphologic and strength differences between eight of the smallest and eight of the largest players competing at the Pee-Wee level of competition (12–13 years) during the 1985–1986 season in Quebec city. The average weight and height differences were 37.2 kg and 31.5 cm, respectively [18]. Furthermore, Bernard et al. [19] found a 357% difference in the force of impact during body checking between the weakest and strongest player participating at the Bantam level of competition (14–15 years) [19].

Suggestions for Injury Prevention

Generally, prevention of injury is multifactorial. Because of the inherent characteristics of ice hockey, injuries are unlikely to be eliminated entirely, regardless of the risk-management strategy employed. Once this is recognized, strategies can be aimed at avoiding unnecessary foreseeable risk, and controlling that which is understood to be inherent to the sport [47]. That said, it is extremely important for sports governing bodies to 'do their homework' prior to introducing new risk management strategies to make sure that preventive strategies do not result in other adverse health effects. Also, once specific actions are taken such as the introduction of a new rule or equipment standard, it is important that sport epidemiologic research continues to assess the effectiveness of the preventative program. Products should be improved and standards changed concurrently with the new experience gained [48].

Protective Equipment

The introduction of mandatory full face shield rules among the pediatric population has dramatically reduced the rate of facial and eye injuries. Until recently, there was controversy that the added protection would increase other injury rates due to a feeling of invincibility leading athletes to take excessive and unwarranted risks. Gerberich et al. [7] found that 66% of high school hockey players from the Minnesota area felt that the requirement of the face mask allowed them to be more aggressive in their style of play. However, data exists in the adult epidemiologic literature to support the protective effect of full face shield use in reducing concussion severity, facial, eye and dental injuries, without increasing other injury rates overall [49, 50]. Whether or not reduced concussion severity with no change in overall injury rates would hold for skeletally immature individuals is not known; however, it would be unethical to find out by putting young athletes at increased risk of injury with the removal of the full face shield. Presently, full face shield use is mandated by all organized Minor hockey associations worldwide.

Mouthguard use has also been mandated by several European amateur leagues, the United States Amateur Hockey Association, High School hockey, Junior hockey, and the Peewee level and higher in Canadian Minor hockey for the purpose of reducing the incidence of dental and concussive head injuries. Although the benefits of mouthguard use in protecting athletes from dental injury is supported in the literature [51–59], controversy exists as to whether mouthguard use can reduce athletes' risk of concussion. The evidence of a protective effect on concussions stemmed primarily from a limited number of case series and retrospective cross-sectional surveys. Some authors have stated that the most important value of mouthguard use in sport is the concussion-saving effect following impact with the mandible [53, 54, 60]. Despite lacking clinical application and study, this notion has influenced decision making regarding mouthguard use in sports. At this stage, there is no valid scientific evidence of an association or lack of association between mouthguard use and reduced concussion risk.

A custom-fitted mouthguard (type III) has been reported to be necessary to ensure retention of the mouthguard in collision or contact sports; the simpler designs do not afford much protection, tend to fit poorly, and often interfere with breathing and speech [61]. An optimal mouthguard thickness of four millimeters at the occlusal surface is recommended [54]. It has been shown that the thickness before and after moulding custom-fitted mouthguards decreases by 25–50% [54]. For type II, or commercial 'boil-and-bite' mouthguards, the thickness decreases by 70–99% at the occlusal surface; this is attributed to a lack of control of pressure exerted by the wearer during fitting [54]. Their advantage lies in their cheap cost and wide-spread availability. The American Society of Testing Materials standard (F697) for the care of mouthguards states that it should be washed in cold or lukewarm soapy water, stored in rigid containers, and replaced when splits appear. In addition, mouthguards should be replaced every 2 years for adults and every 6 months for children up to 16 years of age due to changes in the developing pediatric jaw, including teeth replacement and changes in the size and shape of gums [54].

Anecdotally, suggestions have also been made to improve padding of the shoulder, wrist/hands, and anterior knee, as well as improvements in the helmet, chin strap, and chin piece of full face shields to help further reduce ice hockey injuries to the respective anatomic areas [2, 5, 50].

Rink Demographics

Watson et al. [16] investigated the associations between ice surface size and injuries and aggressive penalties among 328 injured players (16–20 years of age) from 16 teams participating in Canadian Junior hockey. The rates of injury per game were inversely related to ice surface sizes (larger than standard: 0.33, standard: 0.58, smaller than standard: 0.76; p < 0.01). There was no significant association between penalty rates and ice surface. While the standard size of North American arenas has remained constant (200 × 85 ft), there has been an increase in size and speed of players. This presumably leads to greater impact forces between players and with the boards, thereby increasing injury potential. Increasing the ice surface would logically decrease contact between players which may reduce injury rates [16]. In 1989, USA Hockey moved the goal line farther from the end boards in an effort to reduce injuries [34]; whether or not this has in fact led to a decrease in injury rates is not known. In addition, injury rates associated with changes in the material composition of the boards (to facilitate energy absorption) and seamless Plexiglas needs to be investigated [7].

Coaching, Officiating, and Rules

The style of ice hockey has been evolving into a more aggressive sport and illegal actions are evident in every level of competition, ranging from minor hockey to the National Hockey League. The attitude of players needs to focus on fun, skill, and sportsmanship. Although coaches have been shown to believe sportsmanship is very important, only 59% of players aged 9–15 years from 9 minor hockey teams in the Minnesota area believed that sportsmanship was very important, with older players believing it less [15]. Respect for the fellow player must be emphasized in the sport through strict officiating rules which have severe consequences for any individual who deliberately attempts to injure another player through an illegal action such as slashing, checking from behind, high sticking, cross-checking, elbowing, and hits to the head. In addition, referees must maintain strict rule enforcement at all levels of competition to help prevent the release of dangerous mechanical energy exchanges. Because catastrophic injuries most commonly result from illegal play [43], this cannot be overstated. In a published guest editorial, Pashby et al. [62] proposed a 'no head-checking rule' to be implemented in all levels of hockey and in all locations where ice hockey is played to help decrease concussive head injury rates.

Roberts et al. [17] studied game injury rates among 273 high school hockey players from 16 teams competing in an ice hockey tournament and compared the injury rates and penalties assessed under fair-play rules (i.e., competing teams have points added to the tournament point totals for staying under a pre-established limit of team penalties per game) and regular rules. They showed a 4.8:1 ratio of injury rates causing greater than one day time loss, facial lacerations, or concussions among players competing under regular rules versus fair-play rules. In addition, the number of penalties assessed per game averaged 7.1 penalties during fair-play rules and 13 penalties during the regular-rules competition [17].

Whether or not body checking should be allowed at various levels of minor hockey has been a topic of controversy for several years. This stems primarily from size differences between players during the adolescent years when the athlete is vulnerable to epiphyseal injury which has the potential to disrupt growth. In 1976, Quebec and Nova Scotia abolished body-checking for Pee-Wee level players 12 years old and younger [14]. This was soon followed by the provinces of British Columbia, Manitoba, and Ottawa. In 1980, the Canadian Amateur Hockey Association introduced a national rule banning body-checking for all Canadian Pee-Wee hockey players. In 1985, the Canadian Amateur Hockey Association decided to raise all age groups by one year to allow Midget level players (15–16 years) the opportunity to complete high school in their home towns prior to playing junior hockey [14]. With the age change, the Canadian Amateur Hockey Association reconsidered the 'no body-checking' rule, and all provinces with the exception of Nova Scotia allowed body-checking for Pee-Wee players (now 12–13 year olds) for the 1985–1986 season [14].

In 1995, USA Hockey instituted a new rule which made it a penalty if a player completed a check on an opponent who no longer had control of the puck [34]. Another risk management strategy that may effectively reduce injuries in the pediatric population would be to add another referee for games, similar to that introduced by the National Hockey League. Each official could 'patrol' one end of the ice on each side of the red line, catching infractions such as slashing, high sticking, cross-checking, and checking from behind, that might otherwise go unnoticed. This 'extra set of eyes' may also make players more cautious of their actions. Lastly, all official hockey associations should seriously consider mandating all coaches and referees to be certified in basic first aid training before participation. This risk management strategy may help prepare these individuals to more effectively deal with injuries in leagues that do not normally have trained medical personnel readily available.

Injury Surveillance

Validated, comprehensive reporting and recording systems to identify injury trends and potential risk factors associated with injury for players at various levels of amateur hockey is critical so that strategies for prevention and control of injuries may be developed based on evidence. There are several athletic injury reporting systems currently in place. However, it is crucial to be able to compare data from different sources to advance our understanding of athletic injury epidemiology. Meeuwisse and Love [63] reviewed existing athletic injury reporting systems in North America and offered four recommendations to assist in moving toward more universal systems for athletic injury reporting. First, comparability of data between systems should be maximized through clear indication of the reporting system design and the methods of data collection. Secondly, an exact definition should be given as to what constitutes a reportable event (injury). Thirdly, whenever possible, outcome information should be collected on each reported event so that an injury definition may be applied at the time of data analysis. Finally, any limitations or sources of error should be acknowledged [63].

Public Awareness

There has been increasing concern, both public and professional, about the frequency and severity of concussions occurring in ice hockey. The morbidity of severe injuries to the brain is a major public health problem, particularly among the pediatric population, because many athletes who sustain these injuries have persistent symptoms or neuropsychological deficits that result in social dysfunction, lost productivity, and excessive health care costs [64–66]. There is also evidence to suggest that cumulative brain damage may be associated with repeated concussions [64–66].

Social and psychological factors among young hockey players include increased aggressiveness and willingness to take risks, a feeling of invincibility, and a lack of awareness of the possibility of spinal cord injury in hockey [34]. Samuel and Joseph [20] showed that 25% of 103 patients aged 7–18 years presenting to a children's hospital emergency department with a hockey-related injury felt that their equipment made spinal cord injury impossible, and nearly 50% felt that their equipment made brain injury impossible. Furthermore, 32%

of patients stated that they would check illegally to win, and 6% stated that they would purposely injure [20]. Brust et al. [15] showed that only 50% of the 12–15-year-old players studied understood the seriousness of checking another player from behind, and some of them were still willing to do it. Players must be informed of the potential risks of injury associated with collision forces to the head and neck. Intensive educational programs for coaches, players and parents should become an integral part of this sport to facilitate understanding of these risks [7]. Hockey associations should provide information brochures on injury prevention that are based on evidence.

Many cases of cervical spine injuries were the result of illegal pushing or checking from behind [34, 42, 43]. In 1985, the Canadian Amateur Hockey Association introduced specific rules against pushing or checking from behind, and in 1988 a videotape entitled 'Smart Hockey with Mike Bossy' strongly delivered the safety message [34].

Four major 'position/policy statements' regarding player safety in the sport of ice hockey have been put forth by the American Osteopathic Academy of Sports Medicine (2002), the Canadian Academy of Sport Medicine (1988), and Committee on Sports Medicine and Fitness of the American Academy of Pediatrics (2000), respectively. A summary of the recommendations by American Osteopathic Academy of Sports Medicine were as follows:

(1) Education of all hockey personnel, especially players and coaches, of each of the following:
   (a) the potential catastrophic injuries that can occur due to checking from behind, high sticking, and blows to the head, and
   (b) the risk, consequences, and prevention of spinal injury, eye injury, and concussion.
(2) Implementation of the Heads Up Hockey safety program by USA Hockey on a larger scale. The Heads Up Hockey brochure and video should be required reading and viewing for all players aged 19 and under, as well as their coaches.
(3) Mandatory full-face shield protection at all amateur levels.
(4) More extensive research into protective equipment.
(5) Continued research into rink technology, particularly safer boards.
(6) The use of larger ice surfaces, and continued experimentation with 4-on-4 play.
(7) Recognition that checking is an acquired skill that needs to be taught in a developmental fashion by qualified coaches.
(8) Recognition that prevention (by playing clean hockey) is the best strategy, and the most important person to teach this to players is the coach.
(9) A formally scheduled meeting between medical and coaching staff each preseason.

(10) Automatic game suspensions for certain rule violations, including but not limited to checking from behind, violent stick use, blows to the head, and fighting. Suspensions should increase with subsequent violations by the same player [67].

The American Academy of Pediatrics (2000) recommended limiting checking in hockey players 15 years of age and younger as a means to reduce injuries [4]. They also stated that strategies such as the 'fair play concept' may also help decrease injuries that resulted from penalties or unnecessary contact. In addition, the Canadian Academy of Sport Medicine (1988) put forth six recommendations after reviewing the ice hockey injury literature:

(1) A nationwide system for collection and classification of injury data be established.
(2) Body checking be eliminated from levels of minor hockey which are not designed as training for professional and international ranks.
(3) Fighting be completely eliminated from the game of hockey.
(4) A major educational program be undertaken aimed at coaches, trainers, players and parents to deinstitutionalize the current accepted norms of violence and injury.
(5) Increased enforcement of existing rules designed to prohibit unsafe acts is required immediately.
(6) Recreational and old-timer's hockey be brought under regulation to conform to equipment standards for safety [68].

Finally, Canadian Academy Sport Medicine (2000) published a position statement regarding facial protection in ice hockey. Their recommendations were as follows:

(1) All ice hockey participants at all levels wear facial protection. Visors (half face shield) significantly reduce the risk of eye injury, but full facial protection has virtually eliminated facial injury. Referees and linesmen should wear helmets and facial protection which will still allow them to blow the whistle.
(2) Only Canadian Standard Association certified equipment be used.
(3) Equipment must be properly fitted and worn. Helmets should be done up securely (no more than two finger-breadths between the neck and the chin strap). Players should not be allowed to play unless they are wearing their helmet and facial protection appropriately [69].

Suggestions for Further Research

Epidemiologic research contributes to an increased understanding of the incidence and mechanism of injury for specific populations with the ultimate purpose of reducing risk. Specific hockey-related injury risk factors are poorly delineated and rarely studied among pediatric ice hockey players leaving large gaps in the knowledge of appropriate prevention strategies. Potential risk factors for injury must be investigated using sound epidemiological principles to provide credible information [2]. One such example is mouthguard use and concussion risk. Given the world-wide pediatric use of full-face shields providing athletes with dental injury protection, it would be prudent to investigate the potential protective effect of mouthguard use on concussions to determine whether mouthguard use in combination with a full face shield is necessary. In addition, future research should be conducted to determine whether increasing the 'cushioning' of the boards can modify basic qualities of the mechanical energy exchange when a player is checked into the boards, a leading mechanism shown to cause injury in this review. This may help a player's neck decelerate the kinetic energy of their torso after a head-first impact. However, it is important to make sure that this increased 'cushioning' does not decelerate the puck to the point where it no longer rebounds; this may potentially increase player congestion along the boards and subsequently increase injury rates. Furthermore, studies should be conducted to determine whether injury rates can be reduced by increasing athletes' awareness that they are in a vulnerable area for injury, such as a 'danger' line painted approximately 3 feet away from the boards around the circumference of the ice surface or a 'stop sign' on the back of players' jerseys. This could easily be studied in amateur hockey.

Gilder and Grogan [70] studied the effects of strength and conditioning drills on injury rates among junior hockey players and showed that endurance, strength, and power drills can increase the integrity of joints and durability of the muscles to help handle physical contact. Future research should be conducted specifically to determine whether such programs can increase players' resistance to injury.

It is critical that future well-designed, prospective studies of sufficient power incorporate a specific target population, use a strict definition of injury and injury severity, use qualified personnel making the injury diagnoses, and use a validated system of injury surveillance. Accurate athlete-participation (exposure) data measuring each athlete's daily participation, as well as specific risk factor exposure information during practices and games should be collected so that the actual risk of injury associated with a potential risk factor can be determined. This information not only will be important to the athletes' themselves, but crucial for sports governing bodies responsible for player safety and physicians who must provide advice to athletes regarding injury prevention.

References

1 Marchie A, Cusimano MD: Bodychecking and concussions in ice hockey: Should our youth pay the price? Can Med Assoc J 2003;169:124–128.

2 Stuart MJ, Smith A: Injuries in junior A ice hockey: A three-year prospective study. Am J Sports Med 1995;23:458–461.

3 Stuart MJ, Smith AM, Nieva JJ, Rock MG: Injuries in youth ice hockey: A pilot surveillance strategy. Mayo Clin Proc 1995;70:350–356.

4 Committee on Sports Medicine and Fitness, American Academy of Pediatrics: Safety in youth ice hockey: The effects of body checking. Pediatrics 2000;105:657–658.

5 Molsa J, Kujala U, Myllynen P, Torstila I, Airaksinen O: Injuries to the upper extremity in ice hockey: Analysis of a series of 760 injuries. Am J Sports Med 2003;31:751–757.

6 Daly PJ, Sim FH, Simonet WT: Ice hockey injuries: A review. Sports Med 1990;10:122–131.

7 Gerberich SG, Finke R, Madden M, Priest JD, Aamoth G, Murray K: An epidemiological study of high school ice hockey injuries. Childs Nerv Syst 1987;3:59–64.

8 Cantu R: Reflections on head injuries in sport and the concussion controversy (editorial). Clin J Sport Med 1997;7:83 84.

9 Last J: A dictionary of epidemiology. ed 4. 2001, New York, Oxford University Press, Inc.

10 Pinto M, Kuhn J, Greenfield M, Hawkins R: Prospective analysis of ice hockey injuries at the junior level over the course of one season. Clin J Sport Med 1999;9:70 74.

11 Kvist M, Kujala UM, Heinonen OJ, Vuori IV, Aho AJ, Pajulo O, Hintsa A, Parvinen T: Sports-related injuries in children. Int J Sports Med 1989;10:81–86.

12 Bjorkenheim JM, Syvahuoko I, Rosenberg PH: Injuries in competitive junior ice-hockey: 1437 players followed for one season. Acta Orthop Scand 1993;64:459–461.

13 Park RD, Castaldi CR: Injuries in junior ice hockey. Phys Sportsmed 1980;8:81–90.

14 Regnier G, Boileau R, Marcotte G, Desharnais R, Larouche R, Bernard D, Roy MA, Trudel P, Boulanger D: Effects of body-checking in the pee-wee (12 and 13 years old) division in the province of Quebec; in Castaldi CR, Hoerner EF (eds): Safety in Ice Hockey, ASTM STP 1050. Philadelphia, American Society for Testing and Materials, 1989, pp 84–103.

15 Brust JD, Leonard BJ, Pheley A, Roberts WO: Children's ice hockey injuries. Am J Dis Child 1992;146:741 747.

16 Watson RC, Nystrom MA, Buckolz E: Safety in Canadian junior ice hockey: The association between ice surface size and injuries and aggressive penalties in the Ontario hockey league. Clin J Sport Med 1997;7:192–195.

17 Roberts W, Brust J, Leonard B, Hebert B: Fair-play rules and injury reduction in ice hockey. Arch Pediatr Adolesc Med 1996;150:140–145.

18 Roy M, Bernard D, Roy B, Marcotte G: Body checking in pee wee hockey. Phys Sportsmed 1989;17:119–126.

19 Bernard D, Trudel P, Marcotte G, Boileau R: The incidence, types, and circumstances of injuries to ice hockey players at the bantam level (14 to 15 years old); in Castaldi CR, Bishop PJ, Hoerner EF (eds): Safety in Ice Hockey: Second Volume, ASTM STP 1212. Philadelphia, American Society for Testing and Materials, 1993, pp 44–55.

20 Samuel R, Joseph D: Factors associated with significant injuries in youth ice hockey players. Pediatr Emerg Care 1999;15:310 313.

21 Goodman D, Gaetz M, Meichenbaum D: Concussions in hockey: There is a cause for concern. Med Sci Sports Exerc 2001;33:2004–2009.

22 Stuart M, Smith A, Malo-Ortiguera S, Fischer T, Larson D: A comparison of facial protection and the incidence of head, neck, and facial injuries in Junior A hockey players. Am J Sports Med 2002;30:39–44.

23 Smith A, Stuart M, Wiese-Bjornstal D, Gunnon C: Predictors of injury in ice hockey players: A multivariate, multidisciplinary approach. Am J Sports Med 1997;25:500–507.

24 Finke R, Gerberich S, Madden M, Funk S, Murray K, Priest J, Aamoth G: Shoulder injuries in ice hockey. J Orthop Sports Phys Ther 1988;10:54–58.

25   Sutherland G: Fire on ice. Am J Sports Med 1976;4:264–269.
26   de Loes M: Epidemiology of Sports Injuries in the Swiss Organization 'youth and sports' 1987–1989. Int J Sports Med 1995;16:134–138.
27   Montelpare WJ: Final report to the Ontario hockey federation and the Canadian hockey association: Measuring the effects of initiating body checking at the atom age level. 2001, www.bcaha.org/mailouts/2002–07–28/2002–19-Iatt%20Bodychecking%20Report%202002–07–18.pdf.
28   Roberts WO, Brust JD, Leonard B: Youth ice hockey tournament injuries: Rates and patterns compared to season play. Med Sci Sports Exerc 1999;31:46–51.
29   Dryden D, Francescutti L, Rowe B, Spence J, Voaklander D: Epidemiology of women's recreational ice hockey injuries. Med Sci Sports Exerc 2000;32:1378–1383.
30   Castaldi CR: Sports-related oral and facial injuries in the young athlete: A new challenge for the pediatric dentist. Pediatr Dent 1986;8:311–316.
31   Pashby T, Pashby R, Chisholm L, Crawford J: Eye injuries in Canadian hockey. Can Med Assoc J 1975;113:663–666.
32   Pashby T: Eye injuries in Canadian hockey. Phase II. Can Med Assoc J 1977;117:670–678.
33   Pashby T: Eye injuries in Canadian amateur hockey. Can J Ophthalmol 1985;20:2–4.
34   Tator C, Carson J, Edmonds V: New spinal injuries in hockey. Clin J Sport Med 1997;7:17–21.
35   Vinger P, Bentkover J, Sullivan R, Kalin J: The ice hockey face guard: Health care costs and ethics; in Castaldi C, Hoerner E (eds): Safety in Ice Hockey, ASTM STP 1050. Philadelphia, American Society for Testing and Materials, 1989, pp 58–62.
36   Reynen R, Clancy W: Cervical spine injury, hockey helmets, and face masks. Am J Sports Med 1994;22:167–170.
37   Pashby T: Eye injuries in Canadian ice hockey, phase III, older players now most at risk. Can J Ophthalmol 1979;121:643–644.
38   Pashby T: Eye injuries in Canadian amateur hockey: Still a concern. Can J Ophthalmol 1987;22:293–296.
39   Pashby T: Making hockey safer (letter). Can Med Assoc J 1990;142:924.
40   Kelly K, Lissel H, Rowe B, Vincenten J, Voaklander D: Sport and recreation-related head injuries treated in the emergency department. Clin J Sport Med 2001;11:77–81.
41   Tator C, Edmonds V: National survey of spinal injuries in hockey players. Can Med Assoc J 1984;130:875–880.
42   Tator C, Ekong C, Rowed D, Schwartz M, Edmonds V, Cooper P: Spinal injuries due to hockey. Can J Neurol Sci 1984;11:34–41.
43   Tator C, Edmonds V, Lapczak L, Tator I: Spinal injuries in hockey players, 1966–1987. Can J Surg 1991;34:63–69.
44   Tator C, Carson J, Cushman R: Hockey injuries of the spine in Canada, 1966–1996. Can Med Assoc J 2000;162:1–3.
45   Torg J: Epidemiology, pathomechanics, and prevention of athletic injuries to the cervical spine. Med Sci Sports Exerc 1985;17:295–303.
46   Molsa J, Tegner Y, Alaranta H, Myllynen P, Kujala U: Spinal cord injuries in ice hockey in Finland and Sweden from 1980–1996. Int J Sports Med 1999;20:64–67.
47   Clarke KS: Cornerstones for future directions in head/neck injury prevention in sports; in Hoerner EF (ed): Head and Neck Injuries in Sports, ASTM STP 1229. Philadelphia, American Society for Testing and Materials, 1994, pp 3–9.
48   Odelgard B: The development of head, face, and neck protectors for ice hockey players; in Castaldi C, Hoerner E (eds): Safety in Ice Hockey. Philadelphia, American Society for Testing and Materials, 1989, pp 220–234.
49   Benson B, Rose M, Meeuwisse W: The impact of face shield use on concussions in ice hockey: A multivariate analysis. Br J Sports Med 2002;36:27–32.
50   Benson B, Mohtadi N, Rose M, Meeuwisse W: Head and neck injuries among ice hockey players wearing full face shields vs half face shields. JAMA 1999;282:2328–2332.
51   Heintz W: The case for mandatory mouth protectors. Phys Sportsmed 1975;April:61–63.
52   Chapman P: Communication: The bimaxillary mouthguard: Increased protection against orofacial and head injuries in sport. Aust J Sci Med Sport 1985;17:25–29.

53   Chapman P: Orofacial injuries and the use of mouthguards by the 1984 Great Britain rugby league touring team. Br J Sports Med 1985;19:34–36.

54   Chalmers D: Mouthguards: Protection for the mouth in rugby union. Sports Med 1998;25: 339–349.

55   Cummins N, Spears I: The effect of mouthguard design on stresses in the tooth-bone complex. Med Sci Sports Exerc 2002;34:942–947.

56   Mastrangelo F: Eye and face injuries in high school hockey: cutting down the risks; in Castaldi C, Hoerner E (eds): Safety in Ice Hockey, ASTM STP 1050. Philadelphia, American Society for Testing and Materials, 1989; pp 52–54.

57   Labella C, Smith B, Sigurdsson A: Effect of mouthguards on dental injuries and concussions in college basketball. Med Sci Sports Exerc 2002;34:41–44.

58   Ranalli D, Demas P: Orofacial injuries from sport: Preventive measures for sports medicine. Sports Med 2002;32:409–418.

59   Newsome P, Tran D, Cooke M: The role of the mouthguard in the prevention of sports-related dental injuries: A review. Int J Paediatr Dent 2001;11:396–404.

60   Chapman P: Concussion in contact sports and importance of mouthguards in protection. Aust J Sci Med Sport 1985;17:23–27.

61   McCrory P: Do mouthguards prevent concussion? Br J Sports Med 2001;35:81–82.

62   Pashby T, Carson J, Ordogh D, Johnston K, Tator C, Mueller F: Eliminate head-checking in ice hockey. Clin J Sport Med 2001;11:211–213.

63   Meeuwisse W, Love E: Athletic injury reporting. Development of universal systems. Sports Med 1997;24:184–204.

64   NIH consensus development panel on rehabilitation of persons with traumatic brain injury. Rehabilitation of persons with traumatic brain injury. JAMA 1999;282:974–983.

65   Matser E, Kessels A, Lezak MD, Jordan BD, Troost J: Neuropsychological impairment in amateur soccer players. JAMA 1999;282:971–973.

66   Vollmer D, Dacey RJ: The management of mild and moderate head injuries. Neurosurg Clin N Am 1991;2:437–455.

67   Juhn M, Brolinson P, Duffey T, Stockard A, Vangelos Z, Emaus E, Maddox M, Boyajian L, Henehan M: Position statement: Violence and injury in ice hockey. Clin J Sport Med 2002;12:46–51.

68   Canadian Academy of Sport Medicine. Violence and injuries in ice hockey: Position statement. 1988:Gloucester, Ontario.

69   Canadian Academy of Sport Medicine Sport Safety Committee. Use of facial protection in ice hockey. Clin J Sport Med 2000;10:212–213.

70   Gilder K, Grogan J: Prevention of ice hockey injuries by strength and conditioning; in Castaldi C, Bishop P, Hoerner E (eds): Safety in Ice Hockey, ASTM STP 1212. Philadelphia, American Society for Testing and Materials, 1993; pp 56–68.

Dr. Brian Benson c/o Dr. Willem Meeuwisse
Sport Medicine Centre, University of Calgary
2500 University Drive N.W., Calgary, Alberta T2N 1N4 (Canada)
Tel. +1 (403) 220 8426, Fax +1 403 282 6140, E-Mail meeuwiss@ucalgary.ca

Maffulli N, Caine DJ (eds): Epidemiology of Pediatric Sports Injuries: Team Sports.
Med Sport Sci. Basel, Karger, 2005, vol 49, pp 120–139

....

Rugby Injuries

Andrew S. McIntosh

School of Safety Science, the University of New South Wales, Sydney, Australia

Abstract

Objectives: The purpose of this chapter is to review critically the existing studies on
the epidemiology of pediatric rugby injuries and discuss suggestions for injury prevention
and further research. **Data Sources:** Data were sourced from the sports medicine and science literature mainly since 1990, and from a prospective injury surveillance project in
rugby undertaken by the University of New South Wales (UNSW) in Sydney during 2002.
Literature searches were performed using Medline and SportsDiscus. **Main Results:**
Reported injury rates were between 7 and 18 injuries per 1,000 hours played, with the rate of
injuries resulting in loss of playing or training time measured at 6.5–10.6 per 1,000 hours
played. Injury rates increased with age and level of qualification. Head injury and concussion accounted for 10–40% of all injuries. In the UNSW study, concussion accounted for
25% of injuries resulting in loss of playing or training time in the under 13 year age group.
Upper and lower extremity injuries were equally apportioned, with musculoskeletal injuries
being the main type of injury. Fractures were observed in the upper extremity and ankle, and
joint/ligament injuries affected the shoulder, knee and ankle. The tackle was associated with
around 50% of all injuries. The scrum produced fewer injuries, but is historically associated
with spinal cord injury. **Conclusions:** Rugby is a contact sport with injury risks related to
physical contact, primarily in the tackle. Most injuries affect the musculoskeletal system,
with the exception of concussion. Spinal cord injury is rare, but catastrophic. Research is
required to understand better injury risks and to reduce the incidence of shoulder, knee and
ankle joint injuries, concussion and spinal injury.

Introduction

Rugby union football is a popular contact sport played on all continents.
Until 1995, rugby union was an amateur sport, but since then a professional
level has developed. At the professional level, there are major international
competitions such as the Six Nations in Europe, the Tri-Nations between

New Zealand, Australia and South Africa, and the Rugby World Cup. At the 2003 Rugby World Cup, teams from the USA, Canada, Japan, Uruguay, Georgia and Romania participated along with the countries with a stronger rugby tradition. Most rugby participants remain amateur, and one of the great strengths of the code is enthusiastic youth rugby, which is the topic of this chapter.

The objective of this chapter is to review critically the literature on the epidemiology of pediatric rugby injuries. This chapter will examine the incidence, characteristics and determinants of injury and provide practical suggestions for injury prevention and further research. The population studied in the chapter is primarily male school-age players, as there are currently few data on injuries affecting the pediatric female rugby population. Generally, the players studied were no older than 18 years of age. This is an appropriate distinction, as rugby is a popular school sport, and specific laws designed for under 19-year-old players 'depower' the scrum [1]. As some studies refer to youth cohorts, i.e., under 21 years of age, these have also been considered for inclusion.

A literature review was undertaken using Medline and SPORTDiscus. All papers were considered that reported on prospective cohort and cross-sectional studies containing youth rugby populations. In general this meant that most papers reviewed were published after 1990. Papers on specialized topics, e.g. spinal cord injury (SCI) in rugby, were also included.

One of the limitations of the literature is the definition of injury in each study. Definitions ranged from the need for on-field assessment and/or treatment, to attendance at medical stations after the game, to missed games and/or training sessions. Each definition changes the 'injury' characteristics. Inclusion of match injuries will increase the rate, and include more minor soft tissue injuries and concussion. Exclusion of match injuries and a focus on only injuries resulting in loss of playing or training time will bias the injury patterns towards the more serious spectrum of musculoskeletal and neurological injuries.

In addition to the literature review, unpublished data from an ongoing rugby injury surveillance project at the University of New South Wales (UNSW) were extracted to provide a more complete picture, given the relative paucity of published literature on youth rugby. The injury surveillance project at UNSW is examining rugby injury in schoolboys to Australian representative players. For schoolboys participation and injury, data were recorded prospectively in 2002 by trained recorders after obtaining informed consent from the player or his parent/guardian. The recorders attended each game and used standardized injury and participation report forms.

Injury data were analysed for region, nature and cause of injury, athletic exposure measures were calculated, and rates of injury derived. Match injuries and injuries resulting in loss of playing or training time were recorded, but training injuries have not been analysed for this chapter. The data are derived from 67 teams (30 × U18, 19 × U15 and 18 × U13) each participating in an average of 8.6 games in 2002. There was an average of 22.4 participants in each team cohort throughout the season; as substitutes were required due to injury or illness, or player nonselection in the study cohort team.

Incidence of Injury

Injury Rates

Rugby is organised in either interschool or club competitions. Team cohorts are generally based on the age of the player, though some competitions have used body mass criteria, and some retain a 'weigh down' category, whereby lighter players are permitted to play with a younger age group. Teams are graded so that the A team is the most competitive team for the age group. Depending on the school or club size, there may be grades from A to D, and possibly to H. Eleven studies of injuries in youth rugby met the inclusion criteria. Injury rates from these studies and UNSW data are presented in table 1.

Table 1 shows that all but two of the studies reviewed were prospective in design, with a sample period ranging from one season to 30 years [2–12]. Players were aged between 6 and 19 years, but the majority of studies reported on secondary school age players. Davidson [2] collected data over an 18-year period (1969–1986) as School Medical Officer controlling a casualty station for all Saturday interschool rugby matches. During this period, 1,444 school-boys attended the casualty station, with 116 suffering 'severe' injuries. The injury rate was 17.7 per 1,000 hours of match exposure for all injuries, and 1.4 for severe injuries. Sparks [10] analysed data for an even longer period (1950–1979) at the Rugby School, and observed an injury rate of 19.8 injuries per 1,000 hours of match exposure, where an injury resulted in a missed game. This rate was similar to Durie and Munroe's [9] rate of 19.8 for 'minor' injuries. However, other authors observed much lower rates of injuries resulting in loss of playing or training time. For example, Roux et al. [8] observed a rate of 7 injuries per 1,000 hours, and Durie and Munroe's [9] rate of 6.5 for 'moderate' injuries, i.e. those resulting in being unable to play for 1–3 weeks. UNSW data showed a combined rate of 10.6 (CI: 8.3–12.9) injuries resulting in at least one missed game per 1,000 player hours. Reasons for differences in injury rates will be explored later in the chapter, although the different data collection methods and injury definitions play a large role.

The rate of injury increases with age, especially when injuries resulting in loss of playing or training time are considered. Davidson [2] observed that the rate also increased with grade (participation level), so that the injury rate for

Table 1. Summary of injury rates

Study	Design prospective/ retrospective (P) (R)	Data collection	Duration and location	Age group	Number of injuries	Sample size	Rate of injury per 1,000 hours	Other rate of injury
Davidson [2]	P	Attendance at school casualty station on match day	18 years (1969–1986) Sydney Australia	11–19	1,444 presentations 116 severe injuries	Player hours 93,780 player games with 82,107 player hours	17.6/1,000 (all) 1.4 /1,000 (severe)	1.56 per 100 player games 0.12/100 severe
				<13	119	8,750 hours	13.6	
				14 and 15	141	7,675 hours	18.4	
				16>	164	6,410 hours	25.6	
Garraway and Macleod [3]	P	Match and training injuries	1993–1994 season Scotland	under 16	26 injuries to 22 players	204	3.4	
				18–19	72 injuries to 50 players	245	8.67	
Lee and Garraway [4]	P	Match and training injuries	One season: 1993–1994 Edinburgh Scotland	11–19 year olds	154 players with 210 injuries (80% match injuries) 9% severe injury	1,705 players from 9 schools		Total 80.9 injuries per 1,000 player seasons (CI: 68.0–93.9)
Bird [5]	P	Interview	One Season New Zealand			54 boys		6.2 per 100 player games match (CI: 4.7–8.1)
						23 schoolgirls		4.7 per 100 player games (CI: 1.9–9.3)

Table 1 (continued)

Study	Design prospective/ retrospective (P) (R)	Data collection	Duration and location	Age group	Number of injuries	Sample size	Rate of injury per 1,000 hours	Other rate of injury
Pringle [6]	P	Cross section An injury that impaired player performance	Four weeks New Zealand	6–15 year old boys	23	1,932 boys during a 4 week period	15.5	
Bottini [7]	P	Lesion sustained on field during match requiring temporary or permanent substitution	One weekend per season each year from 1991–1997 Argentina	'young' 8–21 years	560	27,253 players		0.021 injuries per player
Roux [8]	P	Structured questionnaire Injury severe enough to prevent the playing returning to rugby for at least 7 days	One Season South Africa	High school students – male	495	26 schools participating in 3,350 games	7 injuries resulting in loss of playing or training time per 1,000 hours	0.7 injuries resulting in loss of playing or training time per 100 player games
Durie and Munroe [9]	P	Match injuries	1998 New Zealand	Boys high school	189 match injured players	23 teams comprising 442 schoolboys in 6,880 player hours	27.5 total 1.7 severe (unable to play >3 weeks)	
Sparks [10]	R	Match injury leading to one missed game	1950–1979 United Kingdom	Rugby school 13–18 year old boys	9,885 injuries	650 players per annum with total of 500,000 hours exposure during 30 seasons	19.8	

Study	R/P	Injury definition	Year / Location	Age group	Injuries	Exposure	Per 1,000 hours match	Per 100 player participations match
Sparks [11]	R	Match injury leading to one missed game	1980–1983 United Kingdom	Rugby school 13–18 year old boys	772 injuries	2,427 players with total of 39,866 hours of match exposure	19.4	
Nathan et al. [12]	P	Injury severe enough to prevent the playing returning to rugby for at least 7 days	1982 South Africa	Schoolboys 10–19 years old	79 injuries (including 50 match injuries)	31 teams participating in 6,075 hours of match exposure and 25,110 hours of training	8.2 match injuries	
UNSW	P	Trained recorders at game	2002 Sydney	U13	65 (8)*	i) 1,570 hours ii) 2,565 participations	41.4** (5.1)***	2.5 (0.3)
				U15	94 (24)	i) 2,325 ii) 2,991	40.4 (10.3)	3.1 (0.8)
				U18	186 (47)	i) 3,535 ii) 4,000	52.6 (13.3)	4.7 (1.2)

*Number of injuries resulting in loss of playing or training time; **the rate of match injuries; ***the rate of injuries resulting in loss of playing or training time.

A and B teams was 24.4/1,000 player hours compared with 20.3 for B and C teams and 9.5 for E–H teams.

Player Position
There are 15 players in arguably 10 distinct positions in a rugby team. These are divided into 8 *forwards* (f) and 7 *backs* (b). In a very general sense, the forwards contest the ball in set plays, such as scrums and line outs, and in general play, e.g. rucks and mauls. In contrast, the backs run with the ball or kick for field position after the ball has been won or retained and recycled by the forwards. Forwards and backs are involved in tackling and defence. Naturally, backs and forwards are involved in ruck and mauls. Davidson [2] observed that the full back (b) was the most frequently injured position, followed by the hooker (f), halves (b) and back row (f). Roux et al. [8] observed a similar pattern, but excluding the hooker and including the wingers (b). Some authors reported that injuries were evenly distributed between forwards and backs for school players [4, 9]. However, shoulder injuries were greater in forwards, and lower limb fractures, in backs [4]. These differences most likely reflect the different periods and geographical locations of the studies.

Injury Characteristics

Injury Onset
The majority of injuries in rugby are acute. No study involved a preseason or ongoing medical screening procedure during the season, so it is difficult to exclude predisposition through asymptomatic injury. While there are a few recurrent injuries reported, these are not classified as overuse or chronic in nature in the published literature. UNSW data indicate that overuse injuries do occur in schoolboys, but they are few.

Injury Location
Table 2 presents the comparison of injury location as a percent of the total number of injuries. A review of table 2 reveals that the greatest proportion of match injuries is to the head, face and neck (range 9.6–44.6%), followed by an even distribution between the upper (range 19.1–35%) and lower extremity (range 23.1–43.4%). Unfortunately, not all published rugby injury studies retained the separation between adults and youths in the calculation of injury region affected. When UNSW injuries resulting in loss of playing or training time are examined, upper and lower extremity injuries become more prevalent, except with under 13 year olds. For under 18 year olds, upper extremity injuries accounted for 23% of match injuries and 36% of injuries resulting in loss of

Table 2. Anatomical location of injury expressed as a percent of total injuries

| | Davidson [2] | Lee and Garraway [4] | Roux et al. [8] | Durie and Munroe [9] | Sparks [10] | Sparks [11] | Nathan et al. [12] | UNSW – Sydney Schools in 2002 | | | | | |
| | | | | | | | | U13 | | U15 | | U18 | |
								Match	Lost time	Match	Lost time	Match	Lost time
Head	14.9							24.6	25.0	17.0	16.7	16.7	19.1
Concussion				2.2	5.2	6.3	25.3	17.0	25.0	16.0	16.7	14.0	19.1
Oro-facial								10.8	0.0	10.6	0.0	17.2	4.3
Neck							12.7	9.2	12.5	7.4	8.3	6.5	4.3
Head and neck	36.6	20.4	29	9.6	16.9	26.8	38	44.6	37.5	35.1	25.0	40.3	27.7
Trunk	6.5	8.1	13	12.2	11.1	10.4	7.6	10.8	0.0	9.6	8.3	8.1	2.1
Upper extremity	27.5	35	20	27.4	25.9	26.5	29.1	20.0	50.0	19.1	20.8	23.1	36.2
Shoulder		9.4		9.6	5.4	4.7		12.3	25.0	12.8	20.8	15.1	23.4
Arm								1.5	0.0	1.1	0.0	1.6	4.3
Elbow				2.6				0.0	0.0	0.0	0.0	0.5	0.0
Forearm								0.0	0.0	2.1	0.0	0.5	2.1
Wrist				4.1				1.5	12.5	1.1	0.0	0.5	0.0
Hand/Fingers				10.7	14.2	16.2		4.6	12.5	2.1	0.0	4.8	6.4
Lower extremities	26.2	31	37	43.4	26.1	36.3	25.3	23.1	12.5	35.1	45.8	26.9	34.0
Pelvis and Hips								3.1	12.5	4.3	4.2	1.6	4.3
Thigh				15.9	9.4	8.1		3.1	0.0	6.4	12.5	4.8	4.3
Knee				7.4	11.0	1.8		6.2	0.0	9.6	4.2	9.7	10.6
Leg				6.3	5.2			3.1	0.0	2.1	0.0	4.3	4.3
Ankle					14.6	7.5		7.7	0.0	8.5	12.5	4.8	8.5
Foot/Toes				13.7	5.9			0.0	0.0	4.3	12.5	1.6	2.1

NB = The fields for head and neck, upper extremity and lower extremity are the totals for those regions. Prevalence data from Lee and Garraway [3] were used to calculate body region distribution.

playing or training time, and for U15s lower extremities went from being 35% of match injuries to 46% of injuries resulting in loss of playing or training time. For these more severe injuries, the shoulder (23%), head (20%), neck (8%), ankle (7%) and knee (5%) account for the greatest proportion of injuries averaged across the 3 age groups.

Situational

Training for rugby can involve skills (individual and team) practice, fitness activities, and contact. The rates of injury for training and match play are different, as training may only involve a small proportion of contested play. Injury rates are lower in training [8, 9, 11]. Durie and Munroe [9] observed that the injury rate at training was 3.4 compared to 27.5 per 1,000 hours in match play. However, 24 and 33% of all moderate and serious injuries, respectively, occurred during training. Bird et al. [5] observed a rate of injury in training of 0.9 per 100 player practices compared with 6.2 per 100 player games, which is comparable with Durie and Munroe [9]. This difference was also observed in other player populations, e.g. seniors and colts.

Rugby football is characterized by contact and noncontact phases, and contested set pieces. The latter include match restarts, scrums and line outs. Contact phases include the tackle, rucks and mauls, and noncontact skills include sprinting, stepping, cutting and kicking. Studies have either analysed injury by phase of play or by cause of injury, leading to different terminologies. For example, knowing that an injury occurred in a ruck does not identify causation, as the injured player might have been struck legally by an opponent in an attempt to drive him off the ball.

Activity

As in other contact sports, the majority of injuries occur during contact. Table 3 shows that in rugby the tackle accounts for the majority of injuries, leading to around 50% of all injuries [4, 8, 10, 11]. Table 3 shows that tackling another player accounted for a greater proportion of injuries (range 5–50%) than being tackled (range 13–32%). In the UNSW study, tackling accounted for 75% of all injuries, resulting in a missed game or training session in the U15s, 63% in U13s and 43% in U18s. Sparks [11] also observed that the tackle was associated with a higher proportion of the more severe injuries. While the proportion of injuries that occurred in rucks, mauls and scrums decreased when the injury outcome was 'more severe', this proportion increased for the tackle and open play.

Roux et al. [8] and Bottini et al. [7] noted that rucking resulted in between 8 and 16% of schoolboy injuries. However, the ruck was not a noteworthy cause of injury in the UNSW study, possibly due to the more prescriptive definitions

Table 3. The injury event. The event leading to injury is expressed as a percent of all injuries

	Lee and Garraway [4]	Bottrin et al [7] U15 to U19 range	Roux et al. [8]	Sparks [11]	Nathan et al. [12]	UNSW – Sydney Schools in 2002					
						U13		U15		U18	
						Match	Lost time	Match	Lost time	Match	Lost time
Tackling another player	40	5 to 11	25	20 (29)*	22	26.2	37.5	33.0	50.0	21.0	23.4
Being tackled	24	13 to 18	30	19 (24)	25	32.3	25.0	22.3	25.0	19.9	19.1
Other/Unknown			7	12 (10)		12.3	12.5	17.0	12.5	15.6	8.5
Other collision or impact with person					18	10.7	12.5	19.2	4.2	29.6	25.5
Scrum collapse or scrum contact	2		8	12 (7)		10.8	0.0	1.1	0.0	4.8	6.4
Overuse						3.1	0.0	2.1	0.0	2.2	6.4
Fall/Stumble on same level						3.1	12.5	1.1	0.0	2.2	2.1
Loose play		30 to 40			11						
Ruck	13	8 to 16	18	19 (14)	6						
Maul		18 to 19		7 (2)							
Foul play			4		8						

*The bracketed figures for 10 are the more severe injuries with 152 injuries from 772 being classified as 'more severe'.

of cause, e.g. struck by player, or changes in the style of rugby. For example, in a ruck or maul the injury might occur when a player is struck by an opponent running into the ruck or maul. Therefore, contact is the primary cause of injury, not the ruck. The nature of rugby is also changing with laws being introduced designed to speed up the 'breakdown', i.e. rucks and mauls. Rugby writers often refer to the differences in northern and southern hemisphere styles of elite level play. These trends might be mimicked by younger players, resulting in differences due to style and law changes. When foul play was measured as an event leading to injury [8, 12], it was observed only to be a minor factor.

Chronometry

Few authors have examined when injuries occur during a game. Durie and Munroe [9] observed that injuries were distributed equally throughout the game, but Sparks [11] found that injury occurrence was greater in the first and fourth quarters of the game. In Bird et al's [5] data, inclusive of other player populations, 46% of game injuries were observed in the first half followed by 40% in the second half, with 14% unknown. Global and regional changes in the management of player substitution, especially over the 50 years encompassed in these two studies, may explain these differences.

Rugby is traditionally a winter sport. The injury rate either decreases during the course of the season [4, 9, 11] or has a bimodal pattern [8, 10] with early and late season peaks. Considering the different climates that rugby is played in, as well as holiday breaks that might occur in mid season, and player preparation, it is difficult to draw any conclusions from these data.

Injury Severity

Injury Type

A review of table 4 shows that sprains and strains accounted for the largest proportion of injury, comprising 24–33% of match injuries and 10–50% of injuries resulting in a missed game or training session. Unfortunately due to the differing terminologies, it is difficult to construct a table using comparable definitions. For example, Bottini et al. [7] observed that 8.2% of injuries were lower limb muscle strains; 11% involved ankle and 4% knee ligament sprain, and 5% were cervical spine sprain/strains. Fractures [2, 4, 8] accounted for between 18 and 27% of all injuries [2, 4, 8]. In the UNSW data, fractures represented only a small percentage of match injuries, 3–8%, but they represented a larger proportion of lost time injury (range 13–21%). These data also demonstrated a trend of increasing risk of fracture with age. Reported rates of joint dislocation were low. The UNSW data indicate that, for the under 15 and

Table 4. Nature of injury as percent of total injuries

	Davidson [2]	Lee and Garraway [4]	Roux et al. [8]	Durie and Munroe [5]	Sparks [10]	Sparks [11]	UNSW – Sydney Schools in 2002					
							U13		U15		U18	
							Match	Lost time	Match	Lost time	Match	Lost time
Sprain/Strain				33.3/~0.4			32.3	12.5	33.0	50.0	24.2	31.9
Superficial		12.2					16.9	37.5	14.9	8.3	18.3	8.5
Intracranial (includes concussion)	14.9		12	2.2	5.2	6.3	16.9	25.0	16.0	16.7	14.0	19.1
Open wound		18.9					6.2	0.0	6.4	0.0	7.0	0.0
Blood injury							1.5	0.0	6.4	0.0	8.6	0.0
Fracture	18	23	27				3.1	12.5	4.3	16.7	7.5	21.3
Dislocation			10				1.5	0.0	2.1	0.0	5.4	0.0

under 18 players, about 25% of all match injuries result in at least one missed game, compared to 12% in the under 13 age group. Therefore, it appears that injury rates and injury severity increase with increasing age.

With regards to severity, Finch et al. [13] noted that 10.9% of hospital accident and emergency presentations due to rugby injuries resulted in hospitalization. This changed the ranking of rugby from tenth, based on accident and emergency presentations, to second, behind cycling, based on the proportion of accident and emergency presentations leading to hospitalization. While the initial ranking is biased due to different levels of participation, Australian football being the code of choice in Victoria, the hospitalization data suggest that comparatively rugby injuries are more severe than other participation sports sampled.

Table 4 shows that concussion/intracranial injury has been observed to account for between 2 and 15% of all injuries in the published data, and 14–17% of the UNSW data. Concussion measurement is confounded by diagnosis [14] and injury sampling, i.e. match injuries need to be observed. No catastrophic head injuries were observed in the UNSW data or in the extended studies of Davidson [2] and Sparks [10, 11]. Apart from concussion, facial and teeth fractures were the most severe injuries to the head. In the UNSW data concussion accounted for 15% of match injuries with the 3 age groups combined and 19% of injuries resulting in loss of playing or training time, although most players returned to match play within 14 days post injury.

There is a range of upper extremity musculoskeletal injuries, with the more severe spectrum including clavicle and forearm fractures, gleno-humeral and acromio-clavicular subluxations or dislocations, and rotator cuff tears. Rates of lower extremity injuries are slightly higher than for the upper limb. Severe lower extremity injuries include knee and ankle ligament injuries, ankle fractures, and tears of the anterior and posterior thigh muscles.

Catastrophic Injury

Even though the overall rate of SCI in rugby is low, there is a distinct SCI risk in rugby unlike many other organised youth sports [15–24]. This injury is associated primarily with the tackle and scrum [15–24]. In a recent review of SCI in Australia between 1986 and 1996 [15], only 6 of the 31 SCI cases occurred in schoolboys, with an annual incidence for schoolboys of 1.7 compared to 4.8 per million adult players for this period. The risk of SCI was 10- to 12-fold greater with adult players than schoolboys [18], an observation supported by Armour et al. [23]. However, reliable exposure data were not available. Injury rates were greater for forwards than backs and occurred in the tackle and scrum.

In the USA during the period 1970–1996, 36 of the 62 cervical spine injuries in rugby occurred in the scrum, including 14 junior players [16, 17].

Considering the whole population, there was a significantly higher risk of SCI on scrum engagement compared with scrum collapse. Scrum-related SCI affected the front row with the hooker, one out of 15 players, suffering 30% of SCI [20]. Noakes et al. [22] reported a 46% reduction in the number of SCIs in schoolboys during the period 1990–1997 in comparison to the period 1963–1989 [21]. The authors postulated that this reduction was due to fewer injuries from high tackles, i.e. above the shoulders, rather than effects of the modified scrum laws that commenced in 1990 to prevent scrum engagement-related SCI. During the 2002 season, the UNSW study observed one odontoid peg fracture without SCI in the schoolboy population, and neck injuries in general accounted for 6% of injuries resulting in loss of playing or training time.

Deaths in schoolboy rugby are rare. In New South Wales since 1994 there have been at least 4 players aged up to and including 20 years who have died while participating in rugby. However, in 3 of these cases the cause of death was a pre-existing disease, e.g. heart disease and asthma [25]. Therefore, participation in sport may have been a contributing factor, but not the cause of death. McCrory et al's [26] study of deaths in football identified 25 cases in the period 1968–1999 in Victoria, Australia. Twenty-two cases occurred in Australian football, and 3 rugby players aged in their forties died. There were 9 cases of intracranial injury resulting from head impacts. Included in the 9 were a 15-, 17- and 19-year-old. In summary, it appears that deaths in rugby are due mainly to pre-existing disease and that the risk may be greater with the 'occasional' player in his late thirties and early forties.

Time Loss

The UNSW data (all ages combined) showed that, while shoulder, ankle and knee injuries accounted for 14, 6 and 9% of all injuries, they accounted for 23, 9 and 8% of injuries resulting in loss of playing or training time, respectively. Thus, prevention and management of shoulder injury requires special consideration. Durie and Munroe [9] observed that, while in total there were 27.5 injuries per 1,000 hours, there were only 1.7 injuries per 1,000 hours that were severe to cause a player to miss 3 weeks.

Injury Risk Factors

Few studies related to youth rugby have tested injury risk factors for their correlation or predictive value. Due to this, it is only possible to report on what is known about injury risks, without the benefit of statistical analyses. In general, contact between players is the main cause of injury in rugby. Around half of the injuries occur in the tackle affecting both the tackler and ball carrier, and producing injuries of all levels of severity. Thus, a review of the activity and injury mechanism at the time of most rugby injuries suggests that improper tackling technique may be an important injury risk factor. While this conclusion may seem obvious, no investigator has yet broken down the game into phases and assessed the rate of injury per phase of play. For example, as there are more tackles than line outs in a game, it is to be expected that more injuries will have occurred during the tackle. In addition, the exact characteristics of tackles that result in injury have not been analysed.

Other risk factors often discussed include team and player size mismatches, the definition of the team cohort, environmental conditions, and padded clothing, such as headgear. With regards to injury risks in elite level Australian football, Norton et al. [27] proposed that many factors, including ground hardness and level of qualification, contributed to higher game speeds and more injury, factors in common with rugby. Therefore, injury risks are most likely multifactorial, requiring extensive research to obtain definitive results. This research is yet to be reported.

Skills

Factors that may give rise to injury risks, including SCI and concussion, in the tackle include: high tackles [22]; high velocity tackles [24]; tackles in which the tackler may have been in the peripheral vision of the ball carrier [24]; 'big hits' [24] in which the ball carrier is tackled by more than one player and/or in a smothering tackle; and a general lack of skill for the tackler [20]. Apart from high tackles and spear tackles, where the ball carrier is speared head first into the ground, the other types of tackle are legal.

The author has recently reviewed the video recordings from 40 games of schoolboy rugby. He observed that, when executing a tackle, the tackler often uses his dominant shoulder irrespective of his position relative to the ball carrier, or is unable to decide which shoulder to use in a front-on tackle. In the latter case, the tackler's head is often the first point of contact with the ball carrier. In either situation, the tackler's head or shoulder is exposed to impact-related injury risks. Injuries to the ball carrier appear to occur due to impact with the opponent/s or during the fall, e.g. falling onto an outstretched arm. The Sydney Morning Herald [28] reported on a case in the United Kingdom in which a boy won £100,000 in 2001 for compensation for injury arising from a tackle.

Change in Rules

The rugby scrum has received substantial attention over the years with regards to SCI. Analysis of scrum engagement lead to law changes to 'depower' this phase in under 19-year-old players. Milburn [29] measured the forces applied to an instrumented scrum machine, and found that the total horizontal forward force on engagement ranged between 4.4 kN for high school players to 8 kN for the Australian national team. After the initial engagement, the sustained force reduced by approximately 20%. The under 19 scrum laws are intended to reduce the engagement force, permit each front row to orient itself well and thus reduce scrum-related injury. There have been no prospective studies to examine whether these laws have been successful, in changing either the biomechanical loads during engagement or injury rates.

Physical Characteristics, Team Cohort and Age

The data presented indicate a trend for increasing injury rates with the age of the player and the level of qualification. While there is much discussion in rugby circles in Australia and New Zealand regarding player and team mismatches due to size, currently no data indicate whether there is a correlation between mismatch and injury. In 2002, a Sydney school's First 15 forfeited games against opponents in its interschool competition due to mismatch, and it is routine procedure for some schools' higher grades to play teams of one to two levels of qualifications lower from a school with a greater depth of grades in an age group. Within any age-based team cohort definition there will be size differences due to genetic and cultural differences, and relative age. Some competitions permit players to 'weigh down' into a younger age group, e.g. U16 to U15, if their weight is below competition agreed thresholds for each age group. A 'weigh down' rule is one mechanism for creating more homogeneous team cohorts and competitions, but it does not address skills, such as the tackle, which appear more important in injury risks.

Suggestions for Injury Prevention

Formal and informal research indicates a number of areas in which the risk of injury in youth rugby could be reduced. However, there are no prospective intervention studies of sufficient size that can provide support for any one specific injury prevention program. Establishing an injury surveillance program is the ideal first step in a program to understand and prevent injury [30]. At the team, club/school and competition level, injury surveillance informs injury risk management.

Due to clear and consistent association between the tackle and injury, the tackle needs to be made safer. Coaching and development of basic skills may make a substantial difference if they reinforce and rehearse (a) body height and the position of the head and shoulder for the tackler, and (b) body posture and falling technique for the ball carrier. Illegal tackles, such as high and spear

tackles, need to be penalised aggressively to discourage this form of dangerous play. On a positive note, safe legal tackling may be a more effective way
of stopping an opponent than unsafe legal tackling. SCI risk may be reduced
through safer tackling and attention on the scrum. The development of training programs for young front rowers and a 'licence' system as they mature
may help to reduce scrum-related injuries through skill development. It
remains to be established whether skill alone or with player physique and
matching of physique in the front row are the determinants of safe scrums.
Scrum training combining live supervised practice and machine practice may
be superior to machine practice alone. An association might exist between
fatigue and diminished scrum technique, although this has not been formally
established.

Padded clothing, including headgear and shoulder pads, has become
popular during the last decade in youth rugby. Research to date [31–34]
indicates that padded headgear does not reduce the incidence of concussion in
schoolboys. Further, the survey responses of under 15 male rugby players [32]
suggested that players believe that they can tackle harder and play more
confidently while wearing headgear. As the action of tackling is responsible for
half of all rugby injuries, this combination of perception and biomechanical
performance is of concern. Research on shoulder pads is even more limited
[35], and the performance of both headgear and shoulder pad is controlled
by the laws of rugby. While shoulder pads have the potential to reduce the
magnitude of the impact force to the chest and shoulders, and thereby decrease
the risk of soft tissue contusions, it is difficult to identify a role in the reduction
of shoulder-related joint or skeletal injury. Mouthguards may reduce the risk of
oro-facial injury, and the few prospective studies generally, but not universally,
confirm this finding [36–38], although in mixed populations.

As in all sports, team and player preparation in the areas of fitness, skills,
knowledge of the laws and understanding of the game are important. An understanding of the game should include awareness of skills that might cause injury
and the known limitations of padded clothing.

Suggestions for Further Research

The immediate research challenge is to establish prospective standardised
injury surveillance projects in youth rugby. Such projects can form the basis of
all other rugby injury research. Unfortunately, environmental and cultural differences may render results from one region difficult to apply into another region.
Research is required into the performance of padded clothing and the interplay
between padded clothing and behavior [39]. While laboratory-based research can

identify ways to improve the performance of padded clothing, such as headgear [40], new designs require formal field evaluation.

The screening of players intrinsically at risk of spinal injury and concussion for physical [41], physiological [42] and, in the latter, neuropsychological indicators [43–46] will become areas of increasing attention over the next decade. This process will determine future return to play guidelines for players post concussion, and guidelines for advising players to cease or not commence rugby due to pre-existing risks of neurological injury.

Research into skills and their role in injury causation will need to become more structured and comprehensive due to the multifactorial nature of injuries. Ethical considerations aside, these studies are expensive and labour intensive. They require the a priori resolution of basic measures such as strength, fitness and skills in children.

An important a challenge is developing mechanisms to inform rugby laws and practice through research.

Acknowledgements

The UNSW injury surveillance study is directed by the author. The investigators are Dr. John Best, Dr. John Orchard and the author. Research assistance was provided by Mr. Trevor Savage, Ms. Maria Romiti and Mr. Cameron French. The study was funded by the Australian Rugby Union and the NSW Sporting Injuries Committee.

References

1   The International Rugby Board and the Australian Rugby Union: Laws of the game of rugby union. Sydney, Australian Rugby Union, ed. 2002.
2   Davidson RM: Schoolboy rugby injuries, 1969–1986. Med J Aust 1987,147.119–120.
3   Garraway M, Macleod D: Epidemiology of rugby football injuries. Lancet 1995;345:1485–1487.
4   Lee AJ, Garraway WM: Epidemiological comparison of injuries in school and senior club rugby. Br J Sports Med 1996;30:213–217.
5   Bird YN, Waller AE, Marshall SW, Alsop JC, Chalmers DJ, Gerrard D: The New Zealand Rugby Injury and Performance Project. Br J Sports Med 1998;32:319–325.
6   Pringle RG, McNair P, Stanley S: Incidence of sporting injury in New Zealand youths aged 6–15 years. Br J Sports Med 1998;32:49–52.
7   Bottini E, Poggi EJT, Luzuriaga F, Secin FP: Incidence and nature of the most common rugby injuries sustained in Argentina (1991–1997). Br J Sports Med 2000;34:94–97.
8   Roux CE, Goedeke R, Visser GR, Van Zyl WA, Noakes TD: The epidemiology of schoolboy rugby injuries. S Afr Med J 1987;71:307–313.
9   Durie RM, Munroe AD: A prospective survey of injuries in a New Zealand schoolboy rugby population. NZ J Sports Med 2000;30:84–90.
10   Sparks JP: Half a million hours of rugby football. Br J Sports Med 1981;15:30–32.
11   Sparks JP: Rugby football injuries, 1980–1983. Br J Sports Med 1985;19:71–75.
12   Nathan M, Goedeke R, Noakes TD: The incidence and nature of rugby injuries experienced at one school during the 1982 rugby season. S Afr Med J 1983;64:132–137.

13   Finch C, Valuri G, Ozanne-Smith J: Sport and active recreation injuries in Australia: Evidence from emergency department presentations. Br J Sports Med 1998;32:220–225.
14   Aubry M, Cantu R, Dvorak J, Graf-Baumann T, Johnston K, Kelly J, Lovell M, McCrory P, Meewisse W, Schamasch P: Concussion in Sport Group. Summary and agreement statement of the First International Conference on Concussion in Sport, Vienna 2001. Recommendations for the improvement of safety and health of athletes who may suffer concussive injuries. Br J Sports Med 2002;36:6–10.
15   Spinecare Foundation and the Australian Spinal Cord Injury Units: Spinal cord injuries in Australian footballers. ANZ J Surg 2003;73:493–499.
16   Wetzler MJ, Akpata T, Laughlin W, Levy AS: Occurrence of cervical spine injuries during the rugby scrum. Am J Sports Med 1998;26:177–180.
17   Wetzler MJ, Akpata T, Albert T, Foster TE, Levy AS: A retrospective study of cervical spine injuries in American rugby, 1970 to 1994. Am J Sports Med 1996;24:454–458.
18   Scher AT: Rugby injuries to the cervical spine and spinal cord: A 10-year review. Clin Sports Med 1998;17:195–206.
19   Scher AT: Catastrophic rugby injuries of the spinal cord: Changing patterns of injury. Br J Sports Med 1991;25:57–60.
20   Quarrie KL, Cantu RC, Chalmers DJ: Rugby union injuries to the cervical spine and spinal cord. Sports Med 2002;32:633–653.
21   Kew T, Noakes TD, Kettles AN, Goedeke RE, Newton DA, Scher AT: A retrospective study of spinal cord injuries in Cape Province rugby players, 1963–1989. S Afr Med J 1991;80:127–133.
22   Noakes TD, Jakoet I, Baalbergen E: An apparent reduction in the incidence and severity of spinal cord injuries in schoolboy rugby players in the Western Cape since 1990. S Afr Med J 1999;89:540–545.
23   Armour KS, Clatworthy BJ, Bean AR, Weels JE, Clarke AM: Spinal injuries in New Zealand rugby and rugby league – A twenty year survey. NZ Med J 1997;110:462–465.
24   Garraway WM, Lee AJ, Macleod DAD, Telfer JW, Deary IJ, Murray GD: Factors influencing tackle injuries in rugby union football. Br J Sports Med 1999;33:37–41.
25   Personal communication with Dr. Johan Duflou, Institute of Forensic Medicine, Glebe, Sydney, Australia.
26   McCrory PR, Berkovic SF, Cordner SM: Deaths due to brain injury among footballers in Victoria, 1968–1999. Med J Aust 2000;172:217–219.
27   Norton K, Schwerdt S, Lange K: Evidence for the aetiology of injuries in Australian football. Br J Sports Med 2001;35:418–423.
28   Sydney Morning Herald: School bans rugby in fear of lawsuits. June 20, 2002.
29   Milburn PD: The biomechanics of rugby scrummaging, University of Wollongong, 1990.
30   van Mechelen W, Hlobil H, Kemper H: Incidence, severity, aetiology and prevention of sports injuries: A review of concepts. Sports Med 1992;14:82–99.
31   McIntosh AS, McCrory P: 'Effectiveness of Headgear in Under 15 Rugby Union Football'. Br J Sports Med 2001;35:167–169.
32   Finch C, McIntosh AS, McCrory P: 'What do under 15 year old schoolboy rugby union players think about protective headgear?'. Br J Sports Med 2001;35:89–94.
33   McIntosh AS, McCrory P: 'Impact energy attenuation performance of football headgear'. Br J Sports Med 2000;34:337–341.
34   Wilson BD: Protective headgear in rugby union. Sports Med 1998;25:333–337.
35   Gerrard DF: The use of padding in rugby union; An overview. Sports Med 1998;25:329–332.
36   Moon DG, Mitchell DF: An evaluation of a commercial protective mouthpiece for football players. J Am Dent Assoc 1961;62:568–571.
37   deWet FA, et al: Mouthguards for rugby players at primary school level. J Dent Assoc S Afr 1981;36:249–253.
38   Blignaut JA, Carsten IL, Lombard CJ: Injuries sustained in rugby by wearers and non wearers of mouthguards. Br J Sports Med 1987;21:5–7.
39   McIntosh AS, McCrory P, Finch C, Chalmers D, Best J: Rugby headgear study. J Sci Med Sport 2003;6:355–359.

40 McIntosh AS, McCrory P, Finch C: Performance enhanced headgear – A scientific approach to the development of protective headgear. Br J Sports Med 2004;38:46–49.
41 Torg JS: Cervical spinal stenosis with cord neurapraxia: Evaluations and decisions regarding participation in athletics. Current Sports Medicine Reports 2002;1:43–46.
42 Jordan B: Genetic susceptibility to brain injury in sports: A role for genetic testing in athletes? Phys Sportsmed 1998;26:25–6.
43 Collie A, Maruff P, Makdissi M, McCrory P, McStephen M, Darby D: CogSport: Reliability and correlation with conventional cognitive tests used in postconcussion medical evaluations. Clin J Sport Med 2003;13:28–32.
44 Maroon JC, Field M, Lovell M, Collins M, Bost J: The evaluation of athletes with cerebral concussion. Clinical Neurosurgery 2002;49:319–332.
45 McCrory P: Treatment of recurrent concussion, Curr Sports Med Rep 2002;1:28–32.
46 McCrory P: When to retire after concussion? Br J Sports Med 2001;35:380–382.

Dr. Andrew S. McIntosh
School of Safety Science
University of New South Wales, Sydney, 2052 (Australia)
Tel. +61 2 9385 5348, Fax +61 2 9385 6190, E-Mail a.mcintosh@unsw.edu.au

Maffulli N, Caine DJ (eds): Epidemiology of Pediatric Sports Injuries: Team Sports.
Med Sport Sci. Basel, Karger, 2005, vol 49, pp 140–169

....
Soccer Injuries

Eric Giza[a], Lyle J. Micheli[b]

[a]Harvard Combined Orthopaedic Surgery Program, Boston, Mass., and
[b]Division of Sports Medicine, Children's Hospital, Boston, Mass., USA

Abstract

Objective: This chapter reviews the existing epidemiological studies on pediatric soccer injuries and discusses possibilities for future research. **Data Sources:** A comprehensive, web-based search of existing soccer injury literature was performed with an emphasis on the pediatric population. The search encompassed all available studies, including European journals and texts, and initial investigations from the 1970s which serve as a basis of comparison to more recent work. **Main Results:** Youth soccer is a relatively safe sport with an injury incidence ranging from 2.3 per 1,000 practice hours to 14.8 per 1,000 game hours. Similar to adults, youth soccer injuries occur mostly in the lower extremities, specifically the knee and ankle. Contusions are the most common injury, and minor/moderate injuries predominate. Extrinsic risk factors for youth soccer include: dangerous play, play on small fields, and inclusion of youth players on adult teams. The most important intrinsic risk factor is the relation of knee injury and female gender. **Conclusions:** Adolescent females suffer a disproportionate number of knee and anterior cruciate ligament injuries compared to adolescent males, but recent injury prevention studies yielded encouraging results. Head injuries in youth soccer are low, and rarely, if ever, occur from head to ball contact. Adherence to the rules of the game, proper coaching, and adequate refereeing are important factors in youth soccer injury prevention.

Introduction

Soccer is the world's most popular organized sport with over 200 million males and 21 million females registered with the Fèdèration Internationale de Football Association (FIFA). There has been a considerable increase in soccer participation by American youth over the past two decades. In 1999, the Soccer Industry Council of America estimated that 18.2 million Americans played organized soccer, with 13.8 million players less than 18 years of age. Among players aged 12–17, participation in soccer rose 20% between 1987 and 1999, and high school participation increased 65% [1–3]. In a comparison of sport participation data from 1983 to 1998, a 159% increase in soccer injuries was evident, indicating a large increase in participation for both boys and girls [4].

Investigations in adult male soccer players identified an incidence of 10–35 injuries per 1,000 game hours [5, 6], and adult female studies revealed an incidence of 2–24 injuries per 1,000 player hours [7–10]. Effectively every player incurs one performance limiting injury per year. However, in a review of 20 epidemiological studies on adult soccer injuries, Dvorak and Junge [5] agreed with Inklaar's [11] conclusion that epidemiological information regarding soccer injuries is inconsistent and far from complete.

FIFA estimates that the average world-wide medical cost of a soccer injury is USD 150, leading to an estimated annual cost of USD 30 billion [5]. In professional English soccer, the average cost due to injury is approximately USD 70 million per season [12]. The rise in youth soccer participation, and the subsequent cost associated with injuries, place an enormous economic pressure on the health care system. The new-found popularity of youth soccer challenges sports medicine professionals to not only identify the injury patterns, but also develop effective treatment and prevention programs. The purpose of this chapter is to review the existing studies on pediatric soccer injuries and discuss possibilities for future research.

A comprehensive, web-based search of the existing soccer injury literature was performed with an emphasis on the pediatric population. The search encompassed all available studies, including some initial investigations from the 1970s which serve as a basis of comparison to more recent work. Some studies which included both adult and pediatric subjects were included due to the paucity of pediatric soccer literature and to provide comparison of the two populations. Case series and case reports were included only if the available literature was sparse, and were not used to discuss injury incidence or risk of injury. Soccer is an international sport, and, although all available English (or English translated) papers were reviewed, the chapter may be limited by the exclusion of foreign studies that were not available on English-based search engines. The method of investigation, and even the definition of an injury, varied widely in the literature, therefore decreasing the validity of direct comparison of some studies.

Incidence of Injury

Soccer has a wide variety of participation levels world-wide, from recreational leagues to international competitions. Even among specific age groups, the skill level and goal of participation is quite diverse. For example, a high school player in the United States may play on a relatively low skilled team while the same 'youth club' player in England could be part of a development program for a well-funded, internationally prominent soccer club. Moreover, within each club there can be different teams such as first team and reserve team.

Participation Level, Age, and Gender

Participation level is an important variable in many studies, but the reader should recognize the limitation of varied terminology between different countries and leagues. The studies from which overall injury rates were determined are summarized in table 1 and grouped into: recreational [13, 14], club [10, 15–23], and mixed (pediatric and adult) [24–27] participation. As seen in table 1, most studies reported the incidence as percentage of total injuries or injuries per number of player hours. Age range is an important factor because many clubs use age to separate teams (10–12-year-old, 14–16-year-old, etc.). In a follow-up study over one season, Schmidt-Olsen found that injury incidence increased with age and older youth players approached the incidence rate in adults (12–13 year olds = 3.4/1,000 h, 14–15 year olds = 3.8/1,000 h, 16–17 year olds = 4.0/1,000 h) [18]. Inklaar et al. [26] also found that, among highly skilled players, the injury rate in 17–18 year olds was higher than in other youth groups. In 2001, Soderman found that 15–17-year-old girls had a higher injury rate than other age groups [10], supporting Maehlum and Daljord's [24] findings in 1984 that most injuries occurred in the female 15–19-year-old age group.

Inklaar et al. [26] also showed that injury rates increase with age and are higher in the adult population compared to youth players. Nilsson and Roaas's [15] findings show a much higher rate for both girls and boys; however, when minor abrasions and blisters were excluded, the injury incidence was similar to other studies (boys = 14.0/1,000 h and girls = 32.0/1,000 h). Both Neilsen and Inklaar found that injury incidence, pattern of injury, and traumatology varied between players at different levels of competition, and that injury rates were higher in more competitive players [25, 26]. In contrast, Peterson et al. [27] colleagues performed a prospective, cohort study that compared soccer injuries at different ages and skill levels. They found that low-level youth players had twice as many injuries as high-level youth players in relation to exposure time.

Although soccer epidemiology studies in the 1970s and early 1980s [15, 19] showed that females had a higher injury rate, age and skill level may have more of an influence on injury incidence than gender alone. In a 5-day invitational tournament in 1985 with over 6,000 players, females aged 17–19 showed a much higher injury rate (47.1/1,000 h) compared to males in the same age group (20.6/1,000 h) [17]. In 1984, Maehlum and Daljord [24] studied injuries at the Norway Cup, one of the world's largest youth club tournaments, and found the

Table 1. A comparison of injury rates in youth soccer

Study, year	Age range (in years)	Design P/R	Data collection I/Q	Duration	Number of injuries	Sample number (number of players unless indicated)	Overall injury rate per 1,000 hours	Game injury rate per 1,000 hours	Practice injury rate per 1,000 hours	Injury rate, other
Recreational										
McCarroll [13], 1984	8–18	P	Q	1 season	176	4,013				4.38%
Backous, 1988	6–17	P	I	5 week camp	216	1,139	8.95			
Club										
Nilsson [15], 1978	11–18	P	I	5 day tournament × 2 years (10 days)	1,534	25,000	Boys = 23.0; Girls = 44.0			
Sullivan [16], 1980	7–18	P	Q	1 season	34	1,272	Boys = 0.51; Girls = 1.1			2.6 per 100 players
Schmidt-Olsen [17], 1985	9–19	P	I	5 day tournament	346	6,600	All = 19.1; Boys = 16.1; Girls = 29.9			
Schmidt-Olsen [18], 1991	12–18	P	Q	1 season	312	495	3.7			
Maehlum [19], 1985	11–18	P	I	6 day tournament	411	1,348 teams	All = 11.7; Boys = 9.9; Girls = 17.6			
Maehlum [20], 1999	9–19	P	I	6 day tournament × 2 years (12 days)	278 (in 1993), 295 (in 1997)		7.7 (in 1993), 7.3 (in 1997)			Boys = 7.6 (in 1993), 6.9 (in 1997); Girls = 8.1 (in 1993), 8.3 (in 1997)
Kibler [21], 1993	12–19	P	I	3 day tournament × 4 years (12 days)	179	480 games	2.38			

Table 1 (continued)

Study, year	Age range (in years)	Design P/R	Data collection I/Q	Duration	Number of injuries	Sample number (number of players unless indicated)	Overall injury rate per 1,000 hours	Game injury rate per 1,000 hours	Practice injury rate per 1,000 hours	Injury rate, other
Junge [22], 2000*	14–18	P	I	1 year	France = 58; Czech = 130	France = 131; Czech = 180		France = 12.7; Czech = 14.8	France = 2.3; Czech = 2.6	
Elias [23], 2001**	9–19	P	I	6 day tournament × 10 years (60 days)	3,840	89,500				Boys = 7.60 (min) – 20.04 (max); Girls = 10.23 (min) – 20.11 (max)
Soderman, 2001	14–19	P	I and Q	1 season	79 (Girls only)	175	6.8	9.1	1.5	
Multiple Age Group										
Maehlum [24], 1984	5–60	R	I	1 year	1,329			Male = 3.3 (all ages); Female = 4.9 (all ages)		
Nielsen [25], 1989	16–adult	P	I	1 season	All ages = 109; Youth = 27	Adult = 93; Youth = 30		High level adult = 18.5; Youth = 14.4	High level adult = 2.3; Youth = 3.6	
Inklaar [26], 1996	13–60	P	Q	1 season	83	Adult = 245; Youth = 232	13–14 years = 12.8; 15–16 years = 16.1; 17–18 years = 28.3			17–18 years and high skill = 34.6; 17–18 years and low skill = 15.7
Peterson [27], 2000	14–adult	P	I	1 year	558	264	16–18 years and high skill = 6.6; 16–18 years and low skill = 13.7			Adult professional = 5.6; Adult amateur = 4.6; Adult club = 20.2

*Study compared youth injuries in France to the Czech Republic (Czech); see text for details.
**Injury rates varied over the 10 years of the tournament maximum (max) and minimum (min) values are show for each gender.

injury rate to be twice as high in girls as boys. In 1999, Maehlum et al. [20] again compared values from the 1984 tournament to the 1993 and 1997 tournaments, and found a 35% total decrease in total injuries with a 50% reduction in female injuries [20]. Elias also found a decline in injury rates for both girls and boys during a large American tournament over a 10-year period [23]. While some studies have shown that youth soccer injury rates are higher in high-skilled players [26], others have shown that low-skilled players are more at risk for injury [27]. High-skilled players train more often and presumably compete more intensely, but poor conditioning and fitness in low-skilled players may lead to more injuries. Comparison of the data in table 1 has shown a narrowing of the injury rate between girls and boys over time, and, if it is presumed that the early injury rates in females are secondary to low skill levels, then the increase in soccer skills and training in girls from the 1980s to 1990s may indicate a relationship between decreased injury and improved soccer skills. Indeed, a study by the FIFA Medical Assessment and Research Centre (FIFA-MARC) in 2002 showed that improved training in low-skilled soccer players can lead to a reduction in injury rates [28].

Player Position

A comparison of injury rates and player position is shown in table 2 [16, 29–31]. Only one study has directly compared injury rates and player position [30]. Accounting for the fact that there are only one or two goalkeepers per team, Junge et al. [30] found that goalkeepers have similar physical and psychological profiles to field players, but a 25% lower injury incidence. There is a specific relationship between injury and player position (table 2), except for Boden's [31] retrospective review of tibia/fibula fractures, who found that forwards suffered nearly 40% of these severe injuries.

Injury Characteristics

Injury Onset

The majority of injuries in youth soccer occur acutely. In a study of adolescent female soccer players, 34% of injuries were chronic [10]. The FIFA-MARC studies of youth soccer injuries revealed that overuse injuries accounted for approximately 18% of injuries and that the number of chronic injuries decreased with a preseason conditioning program [22, 28].

Injury Location

A comparison of anatomical injury location in youth soccer studies is shown in table 3. [10, 13, 15–19, 21–23, 25, 26, 32]. Table 3 shows that the

Table 2. A comparison of injury rates and player position in youth soccer

Study	Age range (in years)	Design P/R	Data collection I/Q	Number of injuries	Sample number (number of players unless indicated)	Goalkeeper (n = number of players unless indicated)	Defender	Midfield	Forward	Unknown position at time of injury
Sullivan [16], 1980	7–18	P	Q	34	1,272	6, 17.6%	11, 32.4%	6, 17.6%	11, 32.4%	
Powell [29], 1999 (Only head injuries)		P	I	Boys = 69; Girls = 76	246 teams	Boys = 11.9%; Girls = 18.8%		Boys (forwards and midfield) = 66.1%	Girls (forwards and midfield) = 70.3%	
Boden [31], 1998 (Only tibia/fibula fractures)	19	R	Q	31	31	2, 6%	6, 19%	5, 19%	13, 42%	5, 16%
Junge [30], 2001	14–18 years, and adults	P	I and Q	GK = 47; F = 511	GK (all) = 28; Field (all) = 236; GK (<18 yrs) = 20; Field (<18 yrs) = 179	All = 6.09; 16–18 and high level = 4.68; 16–18 and low level = 7.46; 14–16 and high level = 3.08; 14–16 and low level = 8.83	Field (all) = 7.42			

Table 3. A comparison of anatomical injury location in youth soccer. All studies are prospective and players are youth club unless indicated. N = player sample, percentage, unless indicated

Author	Nilsson [15]	Sullivan [16]	Schmidt-Olsen [17]	Maehlum [19]	Hoff* [32]	Backous [13]	Nielsen [25]	Schmidt-Olsen [18]	Kibler [21]	Inklaar [26]	Junge** [22]	Elias*** [23]	Soderman [23]
Year	1978	1980	1985	1986	1986	1988	1989	1991	1993	1996	2000	2001	2001
Sample number	25,000	1,272	6,600	1,348 teams	821	1,139	30	496		232	311	89,500	175
Injury site													
Head	54, 10%	5	17, 4.9%	71, 17.3%	O = 10, 22%; I = 6, 8%	7		1.2%	8%			M = 288, 1.56; F = 187, 1.76	
Face								1.9%					
Trunk	37, 7%	1	7, 2.0%	31, 7.5%	O = 4, 8%; I = 11, 5%	8							
Back			6, 1.8%			6		13.8%					1, 1.9%
Abdomen									10.9%				
Upper extremity	80, 15%	5		58, 14.1%	O = 3, 6%; I = 14, 20%							M = 278, 1.51; F = 154, 1.45	2, 3.9%
Shoulder			6, 1.8%					2.6%					
Arm			8, 2.3%					7.7%					
Wrist						4							
Hand			22, 6.3%			6							
Lower extremity				251, 51.0%	O = 26, 63%; I = 43, 58%							M = 1435, 7.79; F = 860, 8.09	

Table 3 (continued)

Author / Year	Nilsson [15] 1978	Sullivan [16] 1980	Schmidt-Olsen [17] 1985	Maehlum [19] 1986	Hoff* [32] 1986	Backous [13] 1988	Nielsen [25] 1989	Schmidt-Olsen [18] 1991	Kibler [21] 1993	Inklaar [26] 1996	Junge** [22] 2000	Elias*** [23] 2001	Soderman 2001
Pelvis/Groin			7, 2.0%			6	4, 14.8%	7.1%			F = 3, 5.3%; Cz = 10, 7.7%		1, 1.9%
Hip Thigh	16, 12%		51, 14.8%			18		1.8%	21%	11	F = 8, 14.0%; Cz = 22, 16.9%	M = 323, 1.65; F = 106, 1.00	14, 26.9%
Knee	72, 14%	4	35, 10.1%			27	6, 22.2%	26%	15.8%	11	F = 14, 24.6%; Cz = 27, 20.8%	M = 348, 1.89; F = 271, 2.55	8, 15.4%
Leg	67, 13%		35, 10.1%			34		10.9%		7	F = 4, 7.0%; Cz = 7, 5.4%	M = 216, 1.56; F = 104, 0.98	3, 5.8%
Ankle	84, 16%	14	55, 15.9%			41	10, 37.0%	23.1%	13%	8	F = 17, 29.8%; Cz = 27, 20.8%	M = 402, 2.18; F = 308, 2.90	18, 34.6%
Foot	67, 13%		97, 28%			22	2, 7.4%	0.3%	12.8%			M = 196, 1.06; F = 86, 0.81	5, 9.6%
Other						37	5, 18.5%	2.2%		6	F = 11, 19.3%; Cz = 36, 7.7%		

*Comparison of outdoor (O) and indoor (I) soccer.
**Comparison of youth soccer injuries in France (F) and Czech Republic (Cz).
***Comparison of male (M) and female (F) injuries. N = injuries, injuries/1,000 player hours.

lower extremity is involved in approximately 60% of injuries, and is the most common injury location in youth soccer. The knee and ankle are the most common sites of injury, in agreement with the adult literature [6, 11, 33, 34]. Upper extremity injuries account for up to 20% of youth injuries, slightly higher than reported for adults [11, 34].

Concussion/Head Injury

Boden et al. [35] determined the incidence of concussion in female collegiate soccer players to be 0.44 per 1,000 athlete exposures; approximately one concussion every 13.5 weeks or one concussion per team per year. The same group also found that 76% of concussions resulted from player-to-player or player-to-object collision (goal post, elbow, sideline advertisement), and only 24% resulted from head-to-ball contact from a ball kicked at full force at a close range [35].

Knee Injuries

The knee can account for up to 25% of all injuries (table 3), similar to adult soccer populations [6, 7, 9, 26, 33, 36–38]. The high incidence of anterior cruciate ligament (ACL) injuries in young female soccer players is alarming. In adults, ACL injury incidence is 0.10 per 1,000 hours, and other investigators found 0.31 adult ACL injuries per 1,000 hours [9, 39].

More adolescent female than male soccer players required ACL reconstruction over a 6-year period at a pediatric sports specialty center [40]. A 1995 study by Arendt and Dick [41] found that female collegiate soccer and basketball players had a significantly higher ACL injury rate than men (0.31 female vs. 0.16 male per 1,000 athlete exposures) [41]. The 1999–2000 National Collegiate Athletic Association injury surveillance data shows the same pattern in young adults and demonstrates that the injury rate is higher in games than practice [42, 43].

Eye Injuries

In a retrospective review of 15 eye injuries which required ophthalmologic consultation, Orlando [44] found hyphema (bleeding within the anterior eye chamber) to be the most common affliction. Six of the fifteen injuries occurred from an underinflated ball which deformed upon striking the head and entered the orbital area.

Wrist Injuries

Upper extremity injuries occur at a much lower frequency than lower extremity injuries (table 3). However, Junge et al. [30] have shown that goalkeepers suffer more upper extremity injuries than field players, but less injuries overall (table 3). In 2001, Boyd et al. [45] prospectively collected data on 1,920 new fractures seen at a pediatric orthopedic center over one year, 29 of which were wrist fractures in youth goalkeepers. They found that a significant number of wrist fractures in children older than 11 years occurred as a result of impact from adult-sized (size five) balls, and suggested that young players should use appropriately sized balls.

Situational Factors

Geographical Region

Injury epidemiology can also vary according to country. In 2000, Junge et al. [22] showed that injury incidence did not vary between youth soccer programs in France and the Czech Republic, but that the number of injuries committed secondary to fouls was higher in the Czech Republic. It is therefore important for the team physician, trainer, or coach to recognize that injury patterns can change in different soccer regions or with different styles of play.

Practice versus Game

A FIFA-MARC study reported that half of youth players consider 'fair fouls' a regular part of the game, and that acceptance of intentional rule violations increases with age and experience [46]. As seen in table 1, youth soccer game injury rates are higher than practice rates [10, 25, 42, 43, 47]. The injury rates reported in tournament-related studies are similar to those for game rates, as tournaments consist primarily of games [15, 17, 19, 23]. Game injury rates are much higher in adults, probably because players will compete more intensely during a match [6, 11, 33, 36].

Indoor versus Outdoor

A comparison of studies with injury data on indoor and outdoor soccer is shown in table 4 [32, 48]. The incidence of indoor soccer injuries in adults has been reported as 4.4 per 100 player hours [49], which is similar to outdoor rates for adults [11, 50]. Indoor soccer has a higher incidence than outdoor soccer due to the smaller playing area, use of walls, and artificial surface [32, 48, 49]. However, only one questionnaire-type study directly compared indoor and outdoor soccer in children [32]. In that study, the incidence of injuries is 4.5 times higher for indoor soccer compared to outdoor soccer, injuries increased with increasing age, and children less than 10 years had relatively few injuries for both indoor and outdoor soccer [32]. Lindenfeld et al. [48] prospectively followed a population of children and adults during one indoor soccer season, and found injury rates similar to outdoor soccer (table 4).

Table 4. A comparison of indoor and outdoor injury rates in youth soccer

Study	Year	Age range (in years)	Design P/R	Data collection I/Q	Duration	Number of injuries	Sample number (number of players unless indicated)	Indoor injury rate per 100 hours	Outdoor injury rate per 100 hours	Practice injuries (number of injuries, percent)	Game injuries (number of injuries, percent)	Injury rate, other
Hoff [32]	1986	8–15	P	Q	1 season	Outdoor = 46; Indoor = 74	Outdoor = 455; Indoor = 366	10.11	5.08	Outdoor = 13, 30.2%; Indoor = 4, 5.5%	Outdoor = 33, (69.8%); Indoor = 70, (94.5%)	
Lindenfeld [48]*	1994	7–50	P	I	7 weeks (adults), 3 weeks (kids)	136 (all)	300 games	All ages = 5.0; <12 yrs: M = 2.8, F = 5.6; 12–15 yrs: M = 4.4, F = 6.3; 16–18 yrs: M = 4.9, F = 4.6				

*Comparison of male (M) and female (F) injuries.

Table 5. A comparison of injury rates and injury mechanism in youth soccer. All studies are prospective unless indicated

Study	Number of injuries	Number of injuries with player contact (N, %, unless indicated)	Number of injuries without player contact (N, %, unless indicated)
Heidt [53]*	Trained = 7; Control = 91	All players = 36, 37%; Trained = 3, 42.9%; Control = 33, 36.3%	All players = 62, 63%; Trained = 7, 57.1%; Control = 55, 63.7%
Junge [22]**	France = 58; Czech = 130	France = 28; Czech = 58	France = 20; Czech = 70
Junge [28]*	Trained = 77; Control = 111	Trained = 0.43 per player per year; Control = 0.74 per player per year[¥]	Trained = 0.34 per player per year; Control = 0.45 per player per year
Kibler [21]	179	56.3%	

*Study involved comparison of group with preseason injury prevention program (Trained) and control group (Control).

**Not all injuries had exact injury mechanism.

[¥]Statistically significant value (p < 0.05) between two groups.

Action or Activity

The outcome of certain injuries is related to the injury mechanism. For example, severe adult ankle injuries are more likely to occur from a contact situation where the foot is planted on the ground [51], while Delfico and Garrett [52] showed that 72% of ACL injuries in soccer occurred from noncontact situations [52]. A comparison of injury mechanisms in youth soccer is shown in table 5 [21, 22, 28, 53]. In the pediatric population, player-to-player contact accounted for approximately half of the injuries [22], and contact occurred in one third of the injuries [53]. Two studies have compared controls to a group of youth players who underwent preseason conditioning [28, 53]. In one study, the control group suffered more injuries due to player-to-player contact, and this could indicate that fitter players are less likely to be hurt during contact situations, such as tackling or heading [28]. In the other investigation, there was no difference in the number of injuries in controls and conditioned players, although this finding may be incidental due to the number of participants [53]. Youth players are most frequently injured during tackles, while professionals are most frequently injured while running. This could indicate that adults or better conditioned adolescents fare better in contact situations [25].

Chronometry
Injury Time During Game/Practice
Drawer and Fuller [12] showed that in professional and World Cup soccer more injuries occur during the second half of a game [6, 33, 37]. In college athletes, a similar game pattern was found, but no relationship to practice time was found [42, 43].

Time of Year
There is a correlation between heat illness and summer soccer tournaments: heat illnesses accounted for 4.5% of injuries in a summer tournament [21]. Elias [23] studied a large summer tournament in Minnesota for over 10 years, and found that the number of heat related illness cases were related to the ambient temperature. Physicians, coaches and trainers should be aware of potential dehydration, and encourage frequent water breaks during summer camps and tournaments [54, 55].

Injury Severity

Injury Type
A summary of studies reporting injury type data is shown in table 6. [10, 13–16, 18, 19, 21, 23, 32, 35, 44, 53, 56, 57] As with adult soccer injury studies [34, 37, 50], contusions represent the most common injury in youth soccer (25–47%). Sprains (20–35%) and muscular strains (8–25%) are also common, and fortunately fractures/dislocations are uncommon and represent approximately 3–12% of injuries reported.

Avulsion Fractures
Rossi and Dragoni [57] reviewed 238 radiographs taken for acute pelvic pain during sports, and found that the prevalence of avulsion fractures in the pelvis in youth soccer is 17.7% (74 of 418 radiographs). The ischial tuberosity was the most common avulsion site (table 6).

Catastrophic Injuries
Fortunately, catastrophic injuries in soccer are rare. A summary of catastrophic injuries in youth soccer is shown in table 7 [58–60]. Death in youth soccer is usually related to falling goalposts. Goalposts rarely fall during the course of normal play, and most accidents related to goalposts are due to climbing or hanging from the goalposts [58, 59]. Goalposts should be properly secured, and the playing field should be cleared of all debris to create a safe environment [60, 61]. In 2003, Filipe et al. [62] outlined the severity and long-term sequelae of 168 eye injuries in soccer. Forty-eight of the 168 injuries occurred among

Table 6. Injury types in youth soccer. All studies prospective unless indicated

Study	Total number of injuries	Abrasion	Contusion	Concussion	Laceration	Fracture/ Dislocation	Pain (site)	Sprain	Strain	Tendonitis/ Inflammation	Other
Nilsson [15]	1,534	336, 39%	306, 36%			29, 3.5%		174, 20% (strains and sprains)			13, 1.5%
Sullivan [16]	34		13, 38.2%			3, 8.8%		12, 35.3%	3, 8.8%		3, 8.8%
McCarroll [14]	176		44, 25.0%	5, 2.8%		22, 12.5%		47, 26.7%	17, 9.7%		41, 23.3%
Hoff [32]*	O = 46; I = 74		O = 8; I = 14			O = 1; I = 7		O = 16; I = 30	O = 11; I = 17		O = 10; I = 6
Maehlum [19]	411		193, 47.0%		74, 18.0%	27, 6.6%		89, 21.7%			28, 6.8%
Backous [13]	216	4	69					35	61	10	37
Schmidt-Olsen [18]	312			1.2%		4%	14% (back)				
Kibler [21]	179		32%	1.5%		9%		21.8%	24.5%		4.5%
Jones [56]**	23					Blow-out fracture = 7					
Inklaar [26]	83		12			2		14	7		
Heidt [53]	98		15			7		25	23	9	8
Elias [23]****	3,840			71, 0.24 per 1,000 h		164, 0.56 per 1,000 h		577, 1.99 per 1,000 h (ankle sprain only)			
Soderman Injury specific studies	79		8			4	19	25	15	3	5

Study	n								
Orlando [44]**	15	Hyphema = 9	Secondary glaucoma = 3	Retinal edema = 5	Corneal laceration = 1	Blow-out fracture = 1	Lid laceration = 1	Angle recession = 5	Chorioretinal rupture = 2
Boden [35]***	29								
Rossi [57]*****	All sports = 203; Soccer = 74	Ischial tuberosity = 34	Anterior inferior iliac spine = 13	Anterior superior iliac spine = 15	Superior corner of pubic symphysis = 6	Iliac crest = 1			

*Comparison of outdoor (O) and indoor (I) soccer.
**Retrospective study including only eye injuries in soccer.
***Investigation of concussions during 2 soccer seasons.
****Not all injury types reported in study.
*****Retrospective study of pediatric pelvic avulsion fractures. All injuries reported represent avulsion fractures.

Table 7. Catastrophic injuries in youth soccer

Study	Total number of injuries	Mechanism	Fatal injuries	Contusion	Concussion	Laceration	Fracture	Cardiac injury	Other	Comment
Blond [58]	117	Falling goalpost	2	40	6	25	37		9	Fatal and severe injury were due to hanging on the goalposts
DeMarco [59]	27	Falling goalpost	18							Goalposts should be secured properly
Stephenson [60]	1	Cranium impaled on fence	1							Fences and debris should be positioned away from playing field

children: Thirty-five were severe (causing permanent visual deficit), and 13 were nonsevere.

Time Loss

A comparison of injury severity in youth soccer is shown in table 8 [10, 16, 21, 22, 28]. The definition of injury and the grading of injury severity varies in the available studies on pediatric soccer injuries. The most widely accepted definition is from Engström et al. [63]. However, the FIFA-MARC has recently modified the definition to include chronic injuries [5, 30] as follows:
(1) Minor Acute: Absence from participation more than one day, but less than one week.
(2) Moderate Acute: Absence from participation of more than 1 week, but less than 4 weeks.
(3) Severe Acute: Absence from participation of more than 4 weeks.
(4) Minor Chronic: Complaint of pain for more than 2 weeks, but less than 4 weeks that does not prevent participation.
(5) Moderate Chronic: Complaint of pain for more than 4 weeks that does not prevent participation.
(6) Severe Chronic (e.g. stress fractures).

Review of the data in table 8 shows that approximately 70–80% of the injuries in youth soccer are minor or moderate, and do not result in a significant loss of time from play. Of 113 severe injuries (both pediatric and adult) that resulted in greater than 4 weeks absence from play, 22.7% occurred in players less than 16 years old, and 25.3% occurred in players aged 16–18 years. Also, the incidence of severe injuries was twice as high in low skilled players compared to highly skilled players [64].

Injury Outcome

An awareness of the propensity for knee injuries in female soccer players is particularly important for the sports medicine professional, as 12 years postinjury, 34% of previous female soccer players in Sweden who suffered an ACL injury have radiographic changes consistent with osteoarthritis [65]. Although there have been no longitudinal studies on the long-term outcome of pediatric soccer injuries, the incidence of hip and knee arthritis for former adult soccer players is much higher when compared to age-matched controls [66, 67].

The relationship of chronic traumatic brain injury and soccer remains a controversial topic, as soccer players exhibit deficiencies in memory and planning compared to controls [68, 69]. In contrast, a recent study used similar neuropsychological tests to those used by Matser et al. [69], and showed that soccer-related concussions were not associated with impaired neurocognitive function [70]. A laboratory study in which a size four ball was lobbed from

Table 8. A comparison of injury severity in youth soccer. All studies are prospective unless indicated

Study	Year	Sample number (number of players unless indicated)	Minor injury	Moderate injury	Severe or major injury
Sullivan	1980	1,272		7	1
Kibler*	1993	74,900 player hours	1st degree = 38%; 1st degree + = 24.5%	2nd degree = 21.8%; 2nd degree + = 7%	3rd degree = 8%; 3rd degree + = 0.6%
Junge**	2000	France = 131; Czech = 180	France = 40.4%; Czech = 40.0%	France = 31.6%; Czech = 35.45%	France = 28.1%; Czech = 24.6%
Soderman**	2001	175	26	41	11
Junge***	2002	Trained = 101; Control = 93	Trained = 0.46; Control = 0.80$^\yen$	Trained = 0.17; Control = 0.24	Trained = 0.14; Control = 0.16

*Moderate = >7 days missed, Severe = season out.
**No clarification of 1st – 3rd degree rating system provided by author.
***Mild ≥1 week loss of participation, Moderate = 2–3 weeks loss of participation, Severe = >4 weeks loss of participation; N = percentage of injuries.
****Minor = 0–7 days absent, Moderate = 7–30 days absent, Major = >30 days absent; N = number of injuries.
¥Statistically significant value (p < 0.05).

three meters found that the greatest peak accelerometer readings had a head injury criteria of only 61, where 1,000 is threshold for brain injury [71]. Naunheim et al. [72] measured head impacts by a triaxial accelerometer placed in a helmet and showed that significantly higher values were reached in soccer than in hockey or football. However, all soccer values were much lower than the impact values needed to cause acute brain injury.

Janda et al. [73] tested the use of padded goalposts in 471 games: no injuries resulted from 7 player/padded post collisions during a 3-year study [73]. They also tested the padded goal posts in the laboratory and showed that the modified posts, even after 2 years of outside exposure, significantly decreased object to post impact force.

Injury Risk Factors

Dangerous Play

Injuries resulting from fouls are potentially preventable injuries. The punishments of a free kick and a yellow or red card for foul tackles are risk control measures that are intended to modify players' behaviors to minimize the number of unsafe acts that expose players to high risk situations. In a study of 4 FIFA tournaments, 63% of tackles that resulted in foot and ankle injuries were deemed to be the result of foul play [51]. Moreover, FIFA [74] specifically declared before the 1998 World Cup competition in France that referees should treat tackles from behind as a foul. Despite this ruling, the proportion of injuries caused by tackles from behind was still high (24%) in the four competitions assessed by Giza et al. [51]. Therefore, youth soccer matches should have adequate refereeing and adhere to the FIFA 'Fair Play' principles [74].

Most concussions are related to collision with another player or the post. Concussions are more likely to occur with rough play, on small fields, and in the penalty area [75].

Age

Soderman [76] found that 59% of females below the age of 16 years playing on senior teams (teams with an average age over 20 years) sustained ACL injuries during contact situations. The authors suggested that female soccer players under the age of 16 years should not be allowed to participate in games at a senior level [76].

Gender

The three to four times higher rate of ACL tear in females compared to males has been attributed to many factors, including joint laxity, core stability, hormonal influence, femoral notch size, and hamstring weakness [9, 77–79]. A recent study in a sheep model by Strickland et al. [80] demonstrated that estrogen did not have an effect on failure of the ACL. However, others have shown an increase in ACL injuries during the ovulatory phase of menstruation [79]. The gender discrepancy in ACL tears appears to be a combination of dynamic factors [78], and there is a low correlation between isokinetic strength measurements and functional tests in adult female soccer players [81].

Level of Play

Elite and professional players achieve a higher level of fitness than recreational players [82], and this fitness level may be protective. Junge et al. [47] have shown a lower injury rate in elite players compared to less skilled players, and a prospective cohort study from the FIFA-MARC showed that the incidence of soccer injuries can be reduced by preventative interventions, especially in low-skill level youth teams [28]. A review of injuries in the elite Women's United Soccer Association by Giza et al. [7] found a relatively low ACL injury rate of 0.09 per 1,000 hours which could represent a 'pre-selection' phenomenon in which players who are at risk for an ACL injury may have had an injury earlier in their career and not reached the Women's United Soccer Association or have had a reconstruction prior to their participation in the Women's United Soccer Association.

Physical Maturity

In 1988, Backous et al. [13] found that boys with the highest incidence of injury were tall (greater than 165 cm) and had a weak grip (less than 25 kg), suggesting that skeletally mature but muscularly weak boys may be more susceptible to injury while playing soccer with peers of the same chronological age.

Suggestions for Injury Prevention

The studies that have addressed injury prevention are summarized in table 9 [28, 53, 71–73, 81, 83, 84]. Review of this table suggests the following preventive measures which are discussed below: shin guards, preseason conditioning, and recognition of physical capabilities.

Shin Guards

While other sports include the use of protective equipment, the main source of protection in soccer is shin guards. Shin guards most likely reduce the incidence of soft tissue injuries, but clinical evidence is lacking. Boden et al. [85] investigated thirty-one fractures of the tibia and fibula in soccer, and found that

Table 9. Suggestions for injury prevention and improved fitness in youth soccer

Study	Year	Design	Purpose	Findings	Conclusions
Junge [28]	2002	Prospective, cohort	Evaluate the effects of a prevention program on the incidence of soccer injuries in male youth amateur players	The prevention group had significantly less players injured (Prevention = 53, Control = 67, p < 0.001) For low skilled players, the prevention group had significantly less injuries per 1,000 player hours (Prevention = 6.95, Control = 11.1, p < 0.05)	The incidence of soccer injuries can be reduced by preventative interventions, especially in low-skill level youth teams
Heidt [53]	2000	Prospective, cohort	Evaluate the role that preseason conditioning had on the occurrence and severity of injury in female soccer players	Less injuries in the preseason training group (Training = 14%, 6 injuries in 42 players; Control = 33.7%, 87 injuries in 258 players)	Preseason conditioning resulted in an overall reduction of injuries to adolescent women playing competitive soccer
Hewett [83]	1999	Prospective, multiple sports	To test the effect of neuromuscular training on the incidence of knee injury in female athletes	97 trained females, 193 untrained females, and 209 male control soccer players were compared 6 severe knee injuries occurred in 5 untrained females and 1 male control No injuries occurred in the trained female group	Decreased incidence of knee injury in female soccer players compared to untrained females utilizing a group of male controls. Subset reported of soccer, but study included basketball and volleyball also

Table 9 (continued)

Study	Year	Design	Purpose	Findings	Conclusions
Janda [73]	1995	Part I: Prospective Part II: Laboratory testing of goalposts	Present laboratory and clinical experience with padded goal posts for preventing head injury in soccer	Padded goal posts significantly decrease object to post impact force in laboratory testing. No injuries resulted from 7 player/padded post collisions during a 3-year study	Subjective questioning of players and coaches revealed did not feel that padded posts negatively effected game play or outcome
Naunheim [72]	2000	Prospective measurements of force in hockey and football, laboratory testing of heading in soccer	To compare acceleration forces to the head in high school-level football, hockey and soccer players	Hockey and football scores from impact during game, but soccer from ball from 30 yards traveling 39 mph Peak *g*'s: Football = 29, Hockey = 35, Soccer = 55	Impacts measured by a triaxial accelerometer placed in a helmet were significantly higher in soccer than in hockey or football; however, all soccer values were much lower than the impact of $200\,g$ needed to cause acute brain injury
Reed [71]	2002	Part I : Eye exam regular play Part II: Field testing of soccer ball to head impact with accelerometer	Define forces of youth soccer heading and determine if it is linked to retinal hemorrhage	After 2 weeks of regular play with an average of 79 headers, eye exams in 21 soccer players were no different than 30 controls With ball lobbed from 3 meters, the mean peak cranial acceleration was 3.7 ± 1.3 Even for greatest impact observed, head injury criteria = 61, where 1,000 is threshold for brain injury	Routine headers not associated with globe impact are unlikely to cause retinal hemorrhage

| Diallo [84] | 2001 | Laboratory testing on group of soccer players and controls | To determine the effects of short-term plyometric training and detraining on motor performance in pubescent soccer players | 10 weeks of specific plyometric training revealed a significant increase in jump, running, and sprint-cycling performances *vs.* controls Results remained after 8 weeks of detraining |
| Ostenberg [81] | 1998 | Laboratory testing on different age groups of female soccer players | Compare isokinetic knee muscle strength, functional performance, aerobic capacity, and general joint laxity between female soccer players >20 years old and <20 years old | Younger players had significantly lower values of isokinetic knee flexor strength, older players had a significantly higher BMI No significant differences for functional performance tests, aerobic capacity, or general joint laxity |

Soccer

90% of players were wearing shin guards at the time of injury, and commented that shin guards are not likely to be helpful after a certain critical force is exceeded. Boden also reviewed the biomechanical studies that have been performed on shin guards and summarized that shin guards decrease the magnitude of forces on the tibia by prolonging the contact time. Depending on the type of shin guard, the load forces were reduced by 41.2–77.1% [31].

Preseason Conditioning

Some authors have shown that preseason neuromuscular training and plyometrics can decrease knee injury rates in females [53, 83, 86]. Heidt et al. [53] evaluated the role that preseason conditioning had on the occurrence and severity of injury in 300 female high school soccer players. The conditioning group of 42 players suffered 6 injuries (one ACL tear), while the control group of 258 players suffered 87 injuries (8 ACL tears) [53]. Hewett et al. [83] performed a prospective cohort study in high school soccer, basketball, and volley ball players in which knee injuries were compared between a preseason conditioned group, a nonconditioned group, and male controls. They found that six severe knee injuries occurred in 5 untrained females and one male control, and that no injuries occurred in the trained female group. Both studies show the positive trends of preventative training, but studies with a large, national injury registry will be needed to statistically prove their effect. In a 3-year prospective study using proprioceptive training for semi-professional soccer players, Caraffa et al. [87] found a significantly lower rate of ACL injury in the trained team compared to the untrained controls [88].

The advent of competitive soccer in the United States has resulted in the opportunity for youngsters to play soccer year round. While increased play can lead to improved skill levels, balance of training is important. Diallo et al. [84] compared a group of 12-year-old boys who underwent a strengthening and fitness program to a control group who only played soccer. They showed that 10 weeks of specific plyometric training resulted in a significant increase in jump, running, and sprint-cycling performances versus controls. They also found that the results remained even after 8 weeks of detraining [84].

Physical Capabilities

The maturation process can also effect the level of play that a soccer athlete achieves. Malina et al. [89] performed a laboratory study on groups of 12-year-old soccer players where height, body mass index, chronological and skeletal age were compared to physical capabilities. They found that elite soccer systematically excludes late maturing boys and favors average and early maturing boys. Reilly et al. [82] have shown that there are anthropometric and physiological predispositions for elite soccer. They state that players may not need to have an extraordinary capacity within any areas of physical performance criteria, but must possess a reasonably high level within all areas, such as muscle strength, aerobic capacity, speed, and coordination. Player position is also related to his or her physiological capacity. Thus, mid-field players and defenders have the highest maximal oxygen intakes and perform best on intermittent exercise tests.

Suggestions for Future Research

Kirkendall and associates at the United States Soccer Federation have commented that, to further our understanding of the relationship between heading, head injury and cognitive deficits, we need to: learn more about the actual impact of a ball on the head, verify the exposure to heading at all ages and competitive levels, determine stable estimates of concussive injury rates across the soccer spectrum, conduct prospective longitudinal studies on soccer players focusing on exposure, injury and cognition, and determine the minimum safe age to begin instruction on the skill of heading [75]. Until the above suggestions can be accomplished, it is important for coaches to teach young soccer players correct heading techniques, such as centering the ball on the forehead, correct timing, and strengthening of the neck muscles. It is also important that parents and coaches are aware of the type of ball used. The balls should be made of a light-weight material that does not readily absorb water during rainy or wet conditions. All young children should use size three balls, and older children should use size four balls. The use of standard size five balls should be reserved for adults and adult-sized teenagers.

Future research should be directed towards longitudinal outcome studies of pediatric soccer injuries to identify those injuries which preclude continuation of the game into adulthood. To accomplish this difficult epidemiological task, injury data surveillance systems will be needed. Currently, comprehensive databases which track injury diagnosis, treatment and outcomes are in place in the National Collegiate Athletic Association and Major League Soccer. Inclusion of these databases by the United States Soccer Federation youth programs is the best model to follow players throughout an established soccer system.

References

1   Metzl JD: Sports-specific concerns in the young athlete: Soccer. Pediatr Emerg Care 1999; 15:130–134.
2   Metzl JD, Micheli LJ: Youth soccer: An epidemiologic perspective. Clin Sports Med 1998; 17:663–673.
3   Soccer Industry Council of America: North Palm Beach, FL 33048: Soccer Industry Council of America; 1999.

4   Jones SJ, Lyons RA, Sibert J, Evans R, Palmer SR: Changes in sports injuries to children between 1983 and 1998: Comparison of case series. J Public Health Med 2001;23:268–271.
5   Dvorak J, Junge A: Football Injuries and Physical Symptoms. Am J Sports Med 2000;28:S3–S9.
6   Hawkins R, Fuller C: A prospective epidemiological study of injuries in four English professional football clubs. Br J Sports Med 1999;33:196–203.
7   Giza E, Mithoefer K, Farrell L, Zarins B, Gill T: Injuries in Women's Professional Soccer. Br J Sports Med 2004. In Print.
8   Engstrom B, Johansson C, Tornkvist H: Soccer injuries among elite female players. Am J Sports Med 1991;19:372–375.
9   Ostenberg A, Roos H: Injury risk factors in female European football. A prospective study of 123 players during one season. Scand J Med Sci Sports 2000;10:279–285.
10 Soderman K, Adolphson J, Lorentzon R, Alfredson H: Injuries in adolescent female players in European football: A prospective study over one outdoor soccer season. Scand J Med Sci Sports 2001;11:299–304.
11 Inklaar H: Soccer injuries I: Incidence and severity. Sports Med 1994;18:55–73.
12 Drawer S, Fuller C: An economic framework for assessing the impact of injuries in professional football. Safety Science 2001;39:in press.
13 Backous DD, Friedl KE, Smith NJ, Parr TJ, Carpine WD Jr: Soccer injuries and their relation to physical maturity. Am J Dis Child 1988;142:839–842.
14 McCarroll J, Meaney C, Sieber J: Profile of Youth Soccer Injuries. Phys Sportsmed 1984;12:113–117.
15 Nilsson S, Roaas A: Soccer injuries in adolescents. Am J Sports Med 1978;6:358–361.
16 Sullivan J, Gross R, Grana W, Garcia-Moral C: Evaluation of injuries in youth soccer. Am J Sports Med 1980;8:325–327.
17 Schmidt-Olsen S, Bunemann LK, Lade V, Brassoe JO: Soccer injuries of youth. Br J Sports Med 1985;19:161–164.
18 Schmidt-Olsen S, Jorgensen U, Kaalund S, Sorensen J: Injuries among young soccer players. Am J Sports Med 1991;19:273–275.
19 Maehlum S, Dahl E, Daljord O: Frequency of injuries in a youth soccer tournament. Phys Sportsmed 1986;14:73–79.
20 Maehlum S, Daljord O, Hansen KJ: Frequency of injuries in youth soccer. Med Sci Sports 1999;31:S401.
21 Kibler W: Injuries in adolescent and preadolescent soccer players. Med Sci Sports Exerc 1993;25:1330–1332.
22 Junge A, Chomiak J, Dvorak J: Incidence of football injuries in youth players. Am J Sports Med 2000;28:S47–S57.
23 Elias SR: 10-year trend in USA Cup soccer injuries: 1988–1997. Med Sci Sports Exerc 2001;33:359–367.
24 Maehlum S, Daljord OA: Football injuries in Oslo: A one-year study. Br J Sports Med 1984;18:186–190.
25 Nielsen A, Yde J: Epidemiology and traumatology of injuries in soccer. Am J Sports Med 1989;17:803–807.
26 Inklaar H, Bol E, Schmikli S: Injuries in Male Soccer players: Team risk analysis. Int J Sports Med 1996;17:229–234.
27 Peterson L, Junge A, Chomiak J, Graf-Baumann T, Dvorak J: Incidence of football injuries and complaints in different age groups and skill-level groups. Am J Sports Med 2000;28:S51–S57.
28 Junge A, Rosch D, Peterson L, Graf-Baumann T, Dvorak J: Prevention of soccer injuries: A prospective intervention study in youth amateur players. Am J Sports Med 2002;30:652–659.
29 Powell JW, Barber-Foss KD: Traumatic brain injury in high school athletes (comment). JAMA 1999;282:958–963.
30 Junge A, Chomiak J, Peterson L, Graf-Baumann T, Dvorak J: Goalkeepers – Physical performance, psychological characteristics and incidence of injuries. Personal Communication 2001.
31 Boden B: Leg injuries and shin guards. Clin Sports Med 1998;17:769–777.
32 Hoff G, Martin T: Outdoor and indoor soccer: Injuries among youth players. Am J Sports Med 1986;14:231–233.

33   Hawkins R, Hulse M, Wilkinson C, Hodson A, Gibson M: The association football medical research programme: An audit of injuries in professional football. Br J Sports Med 2001;35: 43–47.
34   Inklaar H: Soccer injuries II: Aetiology and prevention. Sports Med 1994;18:81–93.
35   Boden B, Kirkendall D, Garrett W: Concussion incidence in elite college soccer players. Am J Sports Med 1998;26:238–241.
36   Dvorak J, Peterson L, Junge A: Risk factors and incidence of injury in football players. Am J Sports Med 2000;28:1–74.
37   Hawkins R, Fuller C: An examination of the frequency and severity of injuries and incidents at three levels of professional football. Br J Sports Med 1998;32:326–332.
38   Ekstrand J, Gillquist J: Soccer injuries and their mechanisms: A prospective study. Med Sci Sports 1983;15:267–270.
39   Bjordal JM, Arnly F, Hannestad B, Strand T: Epidemiology of anterior cruciate ligament injuries in soccer. Am J Sports Med 1997;25:341–345.
40   Micheli LJ, Metzl JD, Di Canzio J, Zurakowski D: Anterior cruciate ligament reconstructive surgery in adolescent soccer and basketball players. Clin J Sport Med 1999;9:138–141.
41   Arendt E, Dick R: Knee injury patterns among men and women in collegiate basketball and soccer NCAA data and review of literature. Am J Sports Med 1995;23:694–701.
42   NCAA. Injury Surveillance System, Men's Soccer. Indianapolis: National Collegiate Athletic Association; 2000.
43   NCAA. Injury Surveillance System, Women's Soccer. Indianapolis: National Collegiate Athletic Association; 2000.
44   Orlando R: Soccer-related eye injuries in children and adolescents. Phys Sportsmed 1988;16: 103–106.
45   Boyd KT, Brownson P, Hunter JB: Distal radial fractures in young goalkeepers: A case for an appropriately sized soccer ball. Br J Sports Med 2001;35:409–411.
46   Junge A: The influence of psychological factors on sports injuries. Am J Sports Med 2000;28: S10–S15.
47   Junge A, Dvorak J, Chomiak J, Peterson L, Graf-Baumann T: Medical history and physical findings in football players of different ages and skill levels. Am J Sports Med 2000;28:S16–S21.
48   Lindenfeld T, Schmitt D, Hendy M, Mangine R, Noyes F: Incidence of injury in indoor soccer. Am J Sports Med 1994;22:364–371.
49   Putukian M, Knowles W, Swere S, Castle N: Injuries in indoor soccer. Am J Sports Med 1996;24:317–322.
50   Dvorak J, Junge A, Chomiak J, Graf-Baumann T, Peterson L, Rosch D, Hodgson R: Risk factor analysis for injuries in football players. Am J Sports Med 2000;28:S69–S74.
51   Giza E, Fuller C, Junge A, Dvorak J: Mechanisms of foot and ankle injuries in soccer. Am J Sports Med 2003;31:550–554.
52   Delfico A, Garrett W: Mechanisms of injury of the ACL in soccer players. Clin Sports Med 1998;17:779–785.
53   Heidt RS Jr, Sweeterman LM, Carlonas RL, Traub JA, Tekulve FX: Avoidance of soccer injuries with preseason conditioning. Am J Sports Med 2000;28:659–662.
54   Casa D, Armstrong L, Hillman S, Montain S, Reiff R, RIch B, Roberts W, Stone J: National Athletic Trainers' Association Position Statement: Fluid replacement for athletes. J Athl Train 2002;35:212–224.
55   Binkley H, Beckett J, Casa D, Kleiner D, Plummer P: National Athletic Trainers' Association Position Statement: Exertional heat illness. J Athl Train 2002;37:329–343.
56   Jones N: Orbital blowout fractures in sport. Br J Sports Med 1994;28:272–275.
57   Rossi F, Dragoni S: Acute avulsion fractures of the pelvis in adolescent competitive athletes: Prevalence, location, and sports distribution of 203 cases collected. Skeletal Radiol 2001;30: 127–131.
58   Blond L, Hansen L: Injuries caused by falling soccer goalposts in Denmark. Br J Sports Med 1999;33:110–112.
59   DeMarco J, Reeves C: Injuries associated with soccer goalposts – United States, 1979–1993. MMWR 1994;43:153–155.

60   Stephenson G, Gibson R: Fatal penetrating head injury during a game of soccer. Injury 1992;23:197–198.
61   Fuller C, Hawkins R: Assessment of football grounds for player safety. Safety Science 1997;2: 115–128.
62   Filipe JC, Fernandes V, Barros H, Falcao-Reis F, Castro-Correia J: Soccer-related ocular injuries. Arch Ophthalmol 2003;121:687–694.
63   Engstrom B, Forssblad M, Johansson C, Tornkvist H: Does a major knee injury definitely sideline an elite soccer player? Am J Sports Med 1990;18:101–105.
64   Chomiak J, Junge A, Peterson L, Dvorak J: Severe injuries in football players. Am J Sports Med 2000;28:S58–S68.
65   Roos H, Ostenberg A, Lohmander L: High prevalence of knee OA and functional limitations in female soccer players with ACL injury. Conference Proceedings: Presentation on female soccer injuries; Gothenburg, Sweden; October 2001.
66   Larsen E, Jensen P, Jensen P: Long term outcome of knee and ankle injuries in elite football. Scand J Med Sci Sports 1999;9:285–289.
67   Lindberg H, Roos H, Gardsell P: Prevalence of coxarthosis in former soccer players. Acta Orthop Scand 1993;64:165–167.
68   Tysvaer AT: Head and neck injuries in soccer. Impact of minor trauma. Sports Med 1992;14: 200–213.
69   Matser E, Kessels A, Lezak M, Jordan B, Troost J: Neuropsychological impairment in amateur soccer players. JAMA 1999;282:971–973.
70   Guskiewicz KM, Marshall SW, Broglio SP, Cantu RC, Kirkendall DT: No evidence of impaired neurocognitive performance in collegiate soccer players. Am J Sports Med 2002;30: 157–162.
71   Reed W, Feldman K, Weiss A, Tencer A: Does soccer ball heading cause retinal bleeding? Arch Pediatr Adolesc Med 2002;156:337–340.
72   Naunheim R, Standeven J, Richter C, Lewis L: Comparison of impact data in hockey, football, and soccer. J Trauma 2000;48:938–941.
73   Janda D, Bir C, Wild B, Olson S, Hensinger R: Goal Post injuries in soccer. Am J Sports Med 1995;23:340–344.
74   FIFA. FIFA Handbook, Laws of the Game. Zurich: FIFA; 1998.
75   Kirkendall DT, Jordan SE, Garrett WE: Heading and head injuries in soccer. Sports Med 2001; 31:369–386.
76   Soderman K, Pietila T, Alfredson H, Werner S: Anterior cruciate ligament injuries in young females playing soccer at senior levels. Scand J Med Sci Sports 2002;12:65–68.
77   Soderman K, Alfredson H, Pietila T, Werner S: Risk factors for leg injuries in female soccer players: A prospective investigation during one out-door season (comment). Knee Surg Sports Traumatol Arthros 2001;9:313–321.
78   Ireland ML: The female ACL: Why is it more prone to injury? Orthop Clin North Am 2002;33: 637–651.
79   Wojtys EM, Huston LJ, Boynton MD, Spindler KP, Lindenfeld TN: The effect of the menstrual cycle on anterior cruciate ligament injuries in women as determined by hormone levels. Am J Sports Med 2002;30:182–188.
80   Strickland S, Belknap T, Turner S, Wright T, Hannafin J: Lack of hormonal influences on mechanical properties of sheep knee ligaments. Am J Sports Med 2003;31:210–215.
81   Ostenberg A, Roos E, Ekdahl C, Roos H: Isokinetic knee extensor strength and functional performance in healthy female soccer players. Scand J Med Sci Sports 1998;8:257–264.
82   Reilly T, Bangsbo J, Franks A: Anthropometric and physiological predispositions for elite soccer. J Sports Sci 2000;18:669–683.
83   Hewett TE, Lindenfeld TN, Riccobene JV, Noyes FR: The effect of neuromuscular training on the incidence of knee injury in female athletes. A prospective study (comment). Am J Sports Med 1999;27:699–706.
84   Diallo O, Dore E, Duche P, Praagh EV: Effects of plyometric training followed by a reduced training programme on physical performance in prepubescent soccer players. J Sports Med Phys Fitness 2001;41:342–348.

85   Boden BP, Lohnes JH, Nunley JA, Garrett WE Jr: Tibia and fibula fractures in soccer players. Knee Surg Sports Traumatol Arthrosc 1999;7:262–266.
86   Silvers HJ, Mandelbaum BR: Preseason conditioning to prevent soccer injuries in young women. Clin J Sport Med 2001;11:206.
87   Caraffa A, Cerulli G, Projetti M, Aisa G, Rizzo A: Prevention of anterior cruciate ligament injuries in soccer. A prospective controlled study of proprioceptive training. Knee Surg Sports Traumatol Arthrosc 1996;4:19–21.
88   Cerulli G, Benoit DL, Caraffa A, Ponteggia F: Proprioceptive training and prevention of anterior cruciate ligament injuries in soccer. J Orthop Sports Phys Ther 2001;31:655–660; discussion 61.
89   Malina R, Reyes MP, Eisenmann J, Horta L, Rodrigues J, Miller R: Height, mass and skeletal maturity of elite Portuguese soccer players aged 11–16 years. J Sports Sci 2000;18:685–693.

Dr. Lyle J. Micheli
319 Longwood Avenue
Boston, MA 02115 (USA)
Tel. +1 508 355 6247, E-Mail mdjenkins@adelphia.net

Maffulli N, Caine DJ (eds): Epidemiology of Pediatric Sports Injuries: Team Sports.
Med Sport Sci. Basel, Karger, 2005, vol 49, pp 170–191

....

Injury Prevention and Future Research

Carolyn A. Emery

Sport Medicine Centre, Faculty of Kinesiology,
University of Calgary, Calgary, Alta., Canada

Abstract

Objectives: To critically examine and summarize the literature identifying risk
factors and prevention strategies for injury in child and adolescent sport. **Data Sources:**
Seven electronic databases were searched including: Medline, Cumulative Index to
Nursing and Allied Health Literature (CINAHL), Psychinfo, Cochrane Database for
Systematic and Complete Reviews, Cochrane Controlled Trials Registry, HealthSTAR and
SPORTDiscus. Medical subject headings and text words included: athletic injury, sport
injury, risk factors, adolescent and child. Additional articles were reviewed based on
sport-specific contributions in the previous chapters of this book. **Main Results:** Despite
the diversity of injuries occurring in various pediatric sporting populations, the unifor-
mity with respect to many of the risk factors identified in the literature is noteworthy (i.e.
previous injury, age, sport specificity, psychosocial factors, decreased strength and
endurance). The literature is significantly limited with respect to the prospective evaluation
of risk factors and prevention strategies for injury in pediatric sport. The consistencies,
however, between the adult and pediatric literature are encouraging with respect to prevention strategies involving neuromuscular training programs (i.e. balance training programs)
to reduce lower extremity injuries in some sports and the use of sport-specific protective
equipment (i.e. helmets). **Conclusions:** Notwithstanding the limitations in the literature,
the successful evaluation of some sport-specific prevention strategies to reduce injury in
pediatric sport is encouraging. There is significant opportunity to methodologically improve
upon the current pediatric sport injury literature in descriptive surveillance research, risk
factor evaluation research, and prevention research. There is a need for prospective studies,
ideally randomized controlled trials, in the evaluation of prevention strategies in pediatric
sport. The integration of basic science, laboratory and epidemiological research is critical in
evaluating the mechanisms associated with injury and injury prevention in pediatric sport.
Finally, long-term studies are needed to identify the public health impact of pediatric sport
injury.

Introduction

Sport injuries in children and adolescents may be predictable and potentially preventable [1, 2]. However, it is impossible to eliminate all injury in youth sport. In some sports, the number and severity of injuries can be reduced through various injury prevention strategies. Though there is less research evidence specifically for the prevention of injuries in youth sport than in adult and elite sport, the impact of sport injury in this population warrants attention.

Participation in physical activity by children and adolescents has important implications for individual and public health benefits. Based on the Canadian Population Health Survey, 65% of adolescents reported participation in regular physical activity at least 12 times per month [3, 4]. For adults, this has decreased significantly to less than 40% of the population over 18 participating in regular physical activity [4]. Similar findings are reported in other countries [5–9]. On average, children 5–12 years spend 18 h per week doing physical activity and youth 13–17 years 15 h per week [3, 4]. This provides ample opportunity for sport injury in this population. Also, 8% of adolescents drop out of recreational sporting activities annually because of injury [8].

Reduction of sport injury would have a major impact on quality of life through the maintenance and promotion of physical activity. There is epidemiological evidence that level of physical fitness is a significant predictor of all-cause mortality, morbidity and disease specific morbidity (i.e. cancer, cardiovascular disease, diabetes) [10–13]. Injuries are also a leading cause for the development of osteoarthritis (OA) in later life. There is evidence that knee and ankle injury, specifically, result in an increased risk of development of OA [14–16]. As such, there is a significant public health impact associated with these injuries and future development of OA and other diseases associated with decreased levels of physical activity. The benefits of sport participation in youth go beyond future health concerns, but also include the benefits of greater self-esteem, relaxation, competition, socialization, teamwork, fitness and greater motor skill development.

A four-stage approach has been proposed to study injury prevention [17]. First, surveillance must be used to measure the extent or magnitude of injury in a given population. Second, causes of injury or risk factors must be identified. Third, prevention strategies need to be developed and validated. Lastly, randomized controlled trials (RCTs) or other intervention studies should be conducted to measure the impact of the prevention strategy, again through surveillance.

Incidence of Injury in Pediatric Sport

Prior to examining potential prevention strategies in child and adolescent sport, we must have a good understanding of the extent of the problem (incidence rates for injury), who is at risk (sport participation), and risk factors for injury in this population. Sport and recreation injuries are a major health problem in Canada and the USA. They represent a leading cause of injury morbidity in many age groups. There is evidence that sports are *the* leading cause of injury requiring medical attention, as well as emergency department admissions, in adolescents [4, 18–20]. Sport injuries account for 50% of all injuries to secondary school children [21]. In Alberta, the reported cumulative incidence rate of adolescent (ages 15–19) sport injuries requiring medical attention is 26 injuries/100 adolescents/year [22]. Sport-specific injury incidence rates exceed this average number in sports such as football, hockey, basketball, wrestling, and gymnastics [5, 20, 22–29]. Studies which have examined only sport injuries reporting to hospital Emergency Departments report rates from 7.03 to 8.55 injuries/100 adolescents/year [18, 30, 31]. Cumulative incidence rates suggest the significance of the public health impact of sport injury. However, they do not take exposure to risk (i.e. hours of participation or number of athlete exposures) into consideration. Increasingly more sport-specific epidemiological studies have included exposure to risk into the study design, and estimate incidence density (i.e. number of injuries/1,000 participation hours or 1,000 athlete exposures) in the results. This facilitates the ability to examine injury risk factors as well as making comparisons across studies.

Acute trauma is one type of injury sustained in child and adolescent sport. In addition, there is growing concern about overuse injury in this population of athletes [32]. This likely reflects increased intensity of training and competition in sport at younger ages, increased skill level at younger ages and longer, often year-round, training seasons [32].

Risk Factors for Injury in Pediatric Sport

Risk factors in sport are any factors which may increase the potential for injury [2]. Risk factors may be extrinsic (i.e. weather, field conditions) or intrinsic (i.e. age, conditioning) to the individual participating in the sport. Modifiable risk factors refer to those which can be altered by injury prevention strategies to reduce injury rates [2, 19]. Nonmodifiable risk factors, which cannot be altered, may affect the relationship between modifiable risk factors and

Table 1. Potential risk factors for injury in child and adolescent sport

Extrinsic risk factors	Intrinsic risk factors
Non-modifiable	*Non-modifiable*
Sport played (contact/no contact)	Previous injury
Level of play (recreational/elite)	Age
Position played	Sex
Weather	
Time of season/Time of day	*Potentially modifiable*
	Fitness level
Potentially modifiable	Preparticipation sport specific
Rules	Training
Playing time	Flexibility
Playing surface (type/condition)	Strength
Equipment (protective/footwear)	Joint stability
	Biomechanics
	Balance/Proprioception
	Psychological/Social factors

injury. Identification of these factors will assist in defining high-risk populations. Potential risk factors are listed in table 1 [1, 19, 33].

Much of the literature addressing child and adolescent sport injury is sport specific and based on descriptive data, which portray primarily the extent of the injury problem. There is a substantial body of literature accumulated over the past decade which demonstrates that risk factors are identifiable for sport- and recreation-related injuries in the adult and elite populations. The evidence for injury prevention strategies reducing the risk of injury in youth sport is weaker and based primarily on cohort studies for specific injuries in specific sports. There is some epidemiological evidence that modifiable risk factors (i.e. decreased levels of sport-specific training in the off-season, endurance, strength and balance) do increase the risk of injury in sports [1, 34–40]. Most of these studies, however, address adult populations and are sport and/or injury specific.

Nonmodifiable Risk Factors for Injury in Pediatric Sport

In identifying nonmodifiable risk factors for injury in child and adolescent sport, there is evidence that males are generally at greater risk for injury (OR = 1.16–2.4) [6, 29, 31, 41–43]. The exception to this is in studies examining specific sports including soccer, baseball, and basketball where females appear to be at greater risk [29, 31, 41–44]. Male children and adolescents participating in sport may generally be at a greater risk of injury as they may be more aggressive, have larger body mass and experience greater contact compared to girls in the same sports. All of these factors may lead to increased forces in running, jumping, pivoting, and contact which may increase susceptibility to injury. In soccer, baseball, and basketball, studies show an increased risk of injury in girls. The reasons for this may be due to lower skill level, or may be of a physiological nature.

Left-handedness also appears to be a risk factor for injury [45]. Left-handed adolescents may be at increased risk of injury because of environmental biases in a right-handed world (i.e. equipment used in sport) or functional differences related to neurological development [45].

Re-injury rates range from 13.1 to 38% [1, 23, 24, 28, 46, 47]. The risk of re-injury in some sports is greater than the risk of first-time injury (RR = 1.35–1.7) [48–50]. Previous injury clearly increases the risk of injury in sport. This finding may be related to persistent symptoms, underlying physiological deficiencies resulting from the initial injury (i.e. ligamentous laxity, muscle strength, endurance, proprioception) and/or inadequate rehabilitation.

Sport-specific rates of injury vary considerably, with the highest rates of injury reported for boys participating in hockey [26, 27], basketball [5, 23, 29] and football [28, 29] and for girls participating in gymnastics [18, 29], basketball [5, 23], and soccer [5, 23, 51]. The lowest rates of injury are consistently reported in swimming, tennis, and badminton [5, 23, 29]. It is not surprising that hockey, basketball, and football are consistently among the top-rated sports for injury in male athletes. There is certainly body contact involved in two of the three sports (hockey and football), and some contact in basketball also. All three sports involve a high rate of jumping, sprinting, and pivoting activity, which are often involved in the mechanism of injury in sport. The findings of Backx et al [5] of outdoor sports, high jump rate sports, and contact sports increasing the risk of injury are consistent with the high rates of injury in these three sports. It is also not surprising that gymnastics, basketball, and soccer are consistently among the top-rated sports for injury in female athletes. These three sports also involve a high rate of jumping, sprinting, and pivoting activities.

The risk of injury consistently increases with age across studies [6, 23, 27–29, 44, 48, 52–59]. In all sports, adolescents (>13 years) are at a greater risk of injury than younger children [6, 23, 27–29, 44, 48, 52–59]. The peak injury rate is consistently in the oldest adolescent age group in youth studies examining all sports, soccer, hockey, football, baseball, and gymnastics [6, 23, 27–29, 44, 55, 59]. Consistency in these findings is not surprising, as level of competition, contact, and size typically increase with age. The time participating in sports likely increases with age and experience. However, exposure-adjusted injury rate (i.e. incidence density) is not always examined.

Injury rates decrease with increasing skill level in hockey [27] and increase with increasing skill level in wrestling and gymnastics [27, 46, 52]. Risk of injury increases with organized sport versus unorganized sport [29], amount of time spent doing sporting activity [42], competition versus practice [37, 52], tournament play versus regular season play [26, 51], increased level of competition [23], indoor versus outdoor soccer [53, 60], and large field size and reduced number of players in Australian Rules football [55]. Injury reporting may be more accurate in studies examining organized sport (i.e. levels of competition) and tournament play accounting for higher injury rates than in unorganized sport. In addition, competitors are more likely to be playing at greater intensity and speeds in competition and tournaments than in practice and regular season play, increasing the risk of sustaining an injury. In Australian Rules football, it is not surprising that larger field size and fewer players (i.e. likely reducing the risk of contact) appear to be associated with a lower risk of injury [55].

There is conflicting evidence regarding anthropometric measurement and risk of injury which appears to be injury and sport specific. Brust et al. [27] demonstrate an increased risk of injury in lighter hockey players with the same age and experience. In football, however, where age categories are also restricted by weight categorization, heavier players are at higher risk of injury than lighter boys [28, 55, 61, 62]. In gymnastics, athletes who are taller or heavier are at an increased risk of injury compared with those shorter or lighter [56, 58, 63]. In soccer, Backous et al. [44] demonstrate that taller players are at an increased risk of injury compared with shorter players. Lyman et al. [54] demonstrate increased risk of elbow symptoms in pitchers who are heavier and taller. Taller and heavier athletes (i.e. in football, gymnastics, soccer, and baseball) may be more susceptible to injury due to greater forces being absorbed through soft tissue and joints. In hockey, a contact sport where there is no weight classification, it is not surprising that the smaller players are more susceptible to injury. Although skeletal maturity may not in itself be a modifiable risk factor, in the context of sport it may be considered modifiable in some sports such as hockey by grouping children by skeletal rather than chronological age.

With rapid skeletal growth occurring in children and adolescents, there are potentially physiological reasons why children and adolescents may be at an increased risk of injury [64]. For example, sudden intense muscular traction exerted on an immature skeleton (i.e. during a period of rapidly increasing muscular strength) may result in an acute avulsion fracture of a growth plate, an injury not possible in adulthood [64]. Chronic repetitive muscular traction exerted on an immature skeleton, usually at the time of a growth spurt, may result in traction apophysitis (i.e. Osgood-Schlatter or Sever's disease) [64]. These are both injuries exclusive to children and adolescents. There is also evidence that there is a noteworthy association between peak height velocity and peak fracture rate of the distal radius, suggesting that a growth spurt may increase the risk of some athletes to some injuries [65].

Potentially Modifiable Risk Factors for Injury in Pediatric Sport
Most studies examining biomechanical alignment, flexibility or strength demonstrate no association of these factors with injury in child and adolescent sport [1, 66–70]. The exceptions to this are found in sport-specific studies. In gymnastics and figure skating there is some evidence of an association between poor flexibility and injury [58, 71]. Both anterior tibiofemoral laxity and pronation are predictive of anterior cruciate ligament knee injury in adolescents [72]. Pasque and Hewett [52] demonstrate an increased risk of shoulder injury in wrestling with increased shoulder ligament laxity. Decreased flexibility is not a risk factor generally for injury in adolescent [1, 69, 70] or adult sport [73]. However, it may be a risk factor for injury in gymnastics, figure skating, and wrestling, all sports that demand a high degree of flexibility for execution of many maneuvers [58, 71].

There is conflicting evidence that elbow injury in baseball pitchers is related to pitching style [68, 74]. Albright et al. [74] found an increased risk of elbow injury with a horizontal arm during delivery (particularly with a whipping or snapping motion) in Little League pitchers (≤14 years). Grana and Rashkin [68] found no relationship between injury and sidearm delivery or speed of delivery in older pitchers (14–19 years). Fatigue based on number of pitches in a game and number of pitches in a season seems to be associated with an increased risk of elbow injury [54]. Fatigue also appears to play a role in hockey where there is an increased risk of injury in the last 5 min of a period and the last period of a game [37]. Lysens et al. [1] report an increased risk of injury in young women with decreased endurance fitness. This is consistent with Cahill and Griffith [40] who found that adolescent football players participating in a prescason conditioning program were at significantly decreased risk of knee injury.

Psychosocial factors may also be potentially modifiable. Faelker et al. [75] demonstrate evidence of a dose-response gradient between decreasing socioeconomic status and increased risk of injury. Studies consistently demonstrate a high correlation between injury in sport and life stress [76–79]. These findings are also consistent with the findings for other injury types (i.e. home, fall, and traffic injury) [75, 78, 79].

Less than 40% of high school rugby participants (n = 2,330) completed any preseason training [80]. High rates of injury may be related to decreased endurance and/or strength associated with limited preseason training, as indicated in both adolescent [1, 40, 53, 81, 82] and adult [35, 36, 83] study findings. Some athlete populations (i.e. low-skill division adolescent female soccer players) may benefit from training programs while others (i.e. high-skill division adolescent female soccer players) may not [81]. Proprioceptive balance training, in conjunction with other training techniques, may reduce the risk of specific injury in specific sport [82–84]. The impact of decreased proprioception as a risk factor for injury remains unclear.

Injury Prevention in Pediatric Sport

As seen throughout sport-specific chapters in this book, as well as in the literature at large, there are very few prospective intervention studies addressing prevention strategies to reduce injury in youth sport. A summary of the prospective intervention studies is shown in table 2 [53, 66, 81, 82, 85–89]. These prevention strategies potentially target risk factors, such as limitations in flexibility, strength, endurance, and proprioception/balance. A nonrandomized prospective intervention study shows no effect of a half-time warm-up and stretching program in high school football [66]. Hewett et al. [85] demonstrate in a nonrandomized prospective study that extensive neuromuscular training programs including flexibility, strength, landing skills, and plyometrics may be effective in reducing injury in adolescent basketball, soccer, and volleyball. In soccer, a significant protective effect of a specific education, conditioning and rehabilitation program in adolescent soccer players is found in the low-skilled division only [RR = 0.63 (95% CI; 0.42–0.94)] [82]. Mykelbust et al. [86] also demonstrate a protective effect of a comprehensive sport-specific balance-training program in the reduction of anterior cruciate ligament injuries in elite adolescent female European handball players in a nonrandomized prospective intervention study. There were only four RCTs identified in a youth population. Emery et al. [87] have demonstrated a protective effect of a home-based balance training program using a wobble board in the reduction of all sport-related injuries in high school physical education participants [RR = 0.2 (95% CI; 0.05–0.88)]. Heidt et al. [53] also demonstrate a protective effect of a multifaceted 7-week preseason training program in female high school soccer players [RR = 0.42 (95% CI; 0.2–0.91)]. Wedderkopp et al. [82] demonstrate a significant reduction of injury in adolescent female European handball with the use of a multifaceted training program which included proprioceptive balance training using a wobble board [RR = 0.17 (95% CI; 0.09–0.32)]. In a further study, they also demonstrate the protective effect of balance board training alone in the reduction of injury in female European handball [RR = 0.21 (95% CI; 0.09–0.53)] [88].

As there are relatively few epidemiological studies addressing modifiable risk factors for injury in child and adolescent sport, it is prudent to discuss

Table 2. Studies examining prevention strategies for injury in child and adolescent sport

Author (year)	Study design (country and time frame)	Participants (age)	Prevention strategy	Injury definition	Results (relative risk = RR, odds ratio = OR, provided adequate information is available)
Bixler and Jones [66] (1992)	Non-RCT (USA)	High school football players (5 teams: 3 intervention, 2 control)	1. Intervention: 1/2 time warm-up and stretching exercises 2. Control: no exercises	Injury requiring medical attention	Injury rates between groups not statistically significant (insufficient data to calculate RR)
Emery et al. [87] (2004)	Cluster RCT (Canada)	120 high school physical education students (14–18) (10 schools)	1. Intervention: daily progressive home program using wobble board 2. Control: no treatment	Injury occurring during a sporting activity which required medical attention and/or loss of at least one day of sporting activity	RR = 0.20 (95% CI; 0.05–0.88) RR (ankle sprain) = 0.14 (95% CI; 0.18–1.13). Multivariate analysis + control for cluster randomization. Greatest effect in those with previous injury. Also demonstrated dose-response effect based on improvements in timed static and dynamic balance.
Heidt et al. [53] (2000)	RCT (USA)	300 female high school soccer players (14–18)	1. Intervention: 7 week preseason Frappier acceleration program (cardio-vascular, plyometrics, strength and flexibility) 2. Control: no preseason program	Injury requiring missing at least 1 game or practice	RR = 0.42 (95% CI; 0.2–0.9)

Study	Type (Country)	Population	Intervention	Outcome	Results
Hewett et al. [85]	Non-RCT (USA)	1,263 high school students (soccer, volleyball and basketball players)	1. Intervention: 366 girls (6-week jump training – 60–90 minutes 3×/week) (includes flexibility, strength, plyometrics, weight training and landing techniques) 2. Control 1: 463 girls 3. Control 2: 434 boys	Serious knee injury (ligament sprain) seen by athletic therapist (>5 days time loss)	14 serious knee injuries (2 intervention, 2 male control, 10 female control) RR = 0.42 (male) RR = 0.17 (female) Significant based on Chi-square analysis (p = 0.05). No control for sport type or factors other than gender
Junge et al. [81] (2002)	Non-RCT (Switzerland)	194 soccer players (mean = 16.5)	1. Intervention: included coach and player education, rehabilitation + conditioning program including cardio-vascular, strength, flexibility and plyometrics training 2. Control: ill-defined	Injury resulting in physical complaint >2 weeks or missed session	1. RR = 0.82 (95% CI; 0.58–1.15) 2. RR (high-skilled divisions) = 0.94 (95% CI; 0.58–1.5) 3. RR (low-skilled divisions) = 0.63 (95% CI; 0.42–0.94)
Marshall et al [89] (2003)	Non-RCT	Little League baseball players (5–18)	1. Reduced-impact safety ball vs. traditional ball 2. Faceguard vs. no faceguard		1. RR (safety ball) = 0.72 (95% CI; 0.57–0.91) 2. RR (faceguard) = 0.65 (95% CI; 0.43–0.98)

Table 2 (continued)

Author (year)	Study design (country and time frame)	Participants (age)	Prevention strategy	Injury definition	Results (relative risk = RR, odds ratio = OR, provided adequate information is available)
Myklebust et al. [86] (2003)	Non-RCT over 3 seasons (60, 58, 52 teams/season) (Norway)	Female European team handball players (16–18)	1. Control year 2. 1st intervention season – floor, balance matt and wobble board exercises (15 min) (handout) – video + coach delivered (3×/week for 5–7 weeks and 1×/week for season) 3. 2nd intervention season – as above but physiotherapist delivered at every practice (15 min) (3×/week for 5–7 weeks and 1×/week for season)	Anterior cruciate ligament injury (>1 week time loss = suspected) as assessed by PT	OR (1st) = 0.87 (95% CI; 0.5–1.52) OR (2nd) = 0.64 (95% CI; 0.35–1.18) OR elite division (2nd) = 0.37 (95% CI; 0.13–1.05)
Wedderkopp et al. [82] (1999)	RCT (Denmark, 1995/96)	237 female European team handball players (16–18)	1. Intervention: practice session training program (warm-up with 2 or more functional large muscle group exercises and proprioceptive ankle disk activity) 2. Control: nonspecific practice session training	Injury requiring player to miss next session or unable to participate without considerable discomfort	RR = 0.17 (95% CI; 0.09–0.32)

| Wedderkopp et al. [88] (2003) | Cluster RCT (Denmark) | 16 teams female European team handball players (16–18) | 1. Intervention: practice session included 10–15 min use of individual ankle disk and warm-up with 2 or more functional large muscle group exercises as in previous study
2. Control group: no ankle disk | Injury requiring player to miss next session or unable to participate without considerable discomfort | OR = 0.21 (95% CI; 0.09–0.53)
Multivariate analysis discomfort but no control of cluster randomization in analysis
Increased risk with increased time in match play |

RCT = randomized controlled trials.

epidemiological evidence in adult sport prior to making recommendations for future research. There is inadequate evidence to support decreased muscle strength, globally, as a risk factor for injury in sport. Emery [34] concludes, based on a systematic review of the literature, that there is evidence of an association between decreased hamstring strength and hamstring strain injury in sport. In a review of the literature, Gleim and McHugh [73] finds no strong evidence that decreased flexibility is associated with injury in sport. There is evidence that decreased sport-specific training in the off-season in professional hockey increased the risk of groin strain injury [RR = 3.38 (95% CI; 1.45–7.92)] [90]. Poor endurance is a risk factor for injury amongst army trainees during the basic training [RR = 2.8 (95% CI; 1.2–6.7) for men and 1.69 (95% CI; 1.2–2.4) for women] [36]. Previous injury appears to be the most significant predictor of sports injury in some studies, with relative risks ranging from 2.88 to 9.41 [17, 35, 84]. Tropp et al. [39] demonstrate that soccer players with functional ankle instability and decreased balance ability were at significantly greater risk of ankle sprain reinjury.

A systematic review of the literature concludes that there are few well-designed studies examining prevention strategies for injury in sport at any age [91]. There are some prospective studies demonstrating the protective effect of equipment in various sports in preventing injury. In baseball and softball, break-away bases reduce sliding injuries significantly [92, 93]. Ankle taping and ankle braces reduce ankle sprain injury in basketball [42, 94]. In ice hockey, full face shields reduce head and face injury [95–98]. Rule modification may also decrease the risk of injuries in some adolescent sports. In football, the elimination of spear tackles significantly reduced the number of head and neck injuries [49, 99]. In ice hockey, fair play rules and making checking from behind illegal significantly reduced overall injury as well as head/neck and back injuries specifically [100, 101]. There is other adult and elite population RCT evidence that balance training in conjunction with other preseason training strategies (i.e. strengthening, endurance training, plyometrics) reduce the incidence of specific injury in specific sports [83, 84, 86, 102–105]. These multifaceted training programs reduce the incidence of ankle sprain injuries and anterior cruciate ligament injuries in some sports. However, balance, endurance, and strength have not been examined as outcome measurements, so it is not clear as to the impact of the training strategies on these potential risk factors.

Protective equipment in many sports (i.e. full face masks and mouth guards in hockey, face shields and safety balls in baseball, shin pads in soccer, helmets in cycling, skiing and snowboarding) exerts a protective effect [89, 95, 106–107]. Regardless, the challenge remains to engage youth in the use of such equipment. Despite the ongoing controversies, educational strategies in combination with legislation or facility/sport association requirements may be the best approach to increasing the use of some protective equipment in some sports.

There is increasing enthusiasm regarding the importance of a preparticipation evaluation by physicians, physiotherapists, and athletic trainers caring for various pediatric athlete populations. The effectiveness of preparticipation evaluation in the prevention of injury in the pediatric population, however, has not been evaluated. Wingfield et al. [108] suggest, based on the results of a systematic review of the literature, that it is difficult to find data to support a specific approach to the preparticipation evaluation or to establish best practices for risk factor identification in any population. As such, standardization of the process is critical prior to attempting to evaluate its effectiveness in any athlete population, including the pediatric population.

Study Limitations in Injury Prevention in Pediatric Sport

To target specific populations of adolescents with those sport-specific training strategies that will have the greatest population health impact; sport participation rates, sports injury rates, and safety behaviors require further examination. Once a specific sport has been targeted for prevention of injury, valid sport injury surveillance systems, including participation exposure and injury data acquisition, require development.

One of the fundamental difficulties in comparing research in sport injury epidemiology is the variability in research design, measurements used to assess exposure and injury, and the variety of risk factors and sports assessed in studies. The research designs reviewed are almost exclusively observational, and intervention studies are not always RCTs. The temporal association between exposure and outcome is often ignored in cross-sectional and case-control studies. For example, Smith et al. [71] examine flexibility in figure skaters already presenting with knee pain, and the temporal association between knee pain and decreased flexibility is unclear.

Injury definition and methods of injury data collection are extremely variable. A major limitation in many studies reviewed is that incidence rates based on number of participants rather than incidence densities based on exposure (i.e. hours or sessions of participation) are used to distinguish high-risk athletes. Clearly, time spent doing an activity is critical in the assessment of risk of injury. Time loss, medical requirements, and reinjury inclusion differ widely between injury definitions. Methods of data collection vary from self-report to therapist or physician report. Only 25–31% of injuries in some studies resulted in a physician consult [5, 23, 24]. Depending on injury definition, some studies may underestimate injury if only those reporting to an emergency room [18, 30, 31, 109], physician, or therapist [37, 51] are included. Other studies may overestimate injury rates if all injuries are reported regardless of reporting source (i.e. parent, coach) [5, 23]. If one relies on self-report, particularly over a longer time frame, incidence rates will likely be underestimated due to recall bias. Bijur et al. [6] demonstrate a 51% increase in self-reported injury over a one-month recall period compared to a 12-month recall period.

Selection bias is of concern in many studies as there is no random selection of participants. Selection bias in which athletes more likely to be injured (i.e. previous injury) and more likely to be in exposure-risk group are selected, may lead to an overestimation of association between risk factor and injury [1, 40, 56, 71, 72, 75, 78, 79, 110]. If there are unreported drop-outs from the study and the reason for drop-out is related to injury, this may lead to an underestimation of association, another form of selection bias. Lack of blinding to exposure status, as with most of the cohort studies examined in this review, may also lead to overestimation of the association.

Poor reliability and validity of exposure measurements (i.e. flexibility, strength) resulting in nondifferential misclassification of exposure (i.e. likelihood of misclassification of exposure is not associated with outcome) will underestimate the association between exposure and injury. This is certainly of concern in studies which demonstrate no association [1, 66, 68–70].

The most noteworthy source of bias in the studies reviewed was a lack of measurement and control for potentially confounding variables. This results most often in an overestimation of association between exposure and injury. When recruitment of subjects is not random, risk factors/training interventions assessed may not be the only difference between groups. Differences in physiological factors, coaching technique, warm-up routines, and equipment may prevail. For example, in Cahill and Griffith's [40] study, a historical cohort, differences attributed to preseason conditioning may be a result of equipment differences, coaching differences, rule changes (i.e. elimination of below the waist blocking in 1973) [111], or physiological factors in the two cohorts, which were not controlled for in the study.

In some RCT studies examining prevention strategies, the intervention was assigned to a team (i.e. cluster), not an individual [53, 81, 82]. If similarities within a team are greater than similarities between teams, these similarities should be controlled for in the analysis (i.e. cluster-adjusted analysis). When clusters are controlled for in an analysis, the effect measure is less precise (i.e. larger 95% CIs) if similarities within each cluster are in fact greater than similarities between clusters [112]. As such, overestimates of the protective effects of training strategies may have been reported as a result of the individual level analyses performed in these intervention studies. In addition, the intervention studies examined identify multifaceted preventative training programs [53, 66, 81, 82]. As a result, it is difficult to identify specific risk factors addressed by the program (i.e. flexibility, strength, endurance, balance) if measurements of these factors are not examined.

External validity of the results in all of the studies examined is limited due to limitations in internal validity. Certainly generalizability beyond the specific sport, age group, level of competition and specific injury type is limited.

In examining Hill's criteria of causation [113], many of the studies reviewed are consistent with the findings in adult population studies. The strength of the associations found between preparticipation training programs and injury are convincing based on the magnitude of the associations found, despite concerns with internal validity and individual level analysis. Specificity, implying that a specific cause leads to a specific effect is difficult to identify when studies often do not control for other risk factors, and injury outcome is often global and poorly defined. Temporal association is clear only in the cohort studies and RCTs reviewed. The only studies providing a clear indication of a dose-response relationship are Faelker's [75], in which injury rate increases with increasing level of poverty and the studies examining increased risk of injury with increasing age [6, 23, 28, 48, 54, 56]. Biological plausibility of risk factors and coherence to existing knowledge has been discussed. Injury prevention studies are few, thus experimental evidence is limited.

Conclusions and Future Research in Injury Prevention in Pediatric Sport

Child and adolescent participation rates in sport are high. High rates of sport injury in this population have a substantial impact on the individual, their parents, and the health care system. Sport injury in children and adolescents may also potentially affect future involvement in physical activity and the future health of our population.

The strength of the evidence for potentially modifiable risk factors for injury in children and adolescents is limited by research design and concerns with internal validity. In case-control and cross-sectional study designs, the temporal association between exposure and outcome is unclear. In many of the cohort studies and nonrandomized intervention studies reviewed, various sources of bias in the selection of subjects, measurement of exposure and outcome variables and lack of control for other potentially confounding variables threaten the internal validity of the studies. There is limited RCT evidence supporting preventative training programs in specific sports in adolescents to reduce the risk of injury. There is more convincing evidence in adult epidemiological studies that decreased endurance, decreased strength, decreased balance, and decreased preseason sport-specific training are associated with sports injury. The consistency of the findings between child and adolescent studies reviewed and the adult population studies is encouraging.

Given the limited number of prospective studies found in the pediatric sport injury literature, it is very likely that other risk factors have not been identified to date, much less evaluated adequately. For example, it is possible that coaching factors (i.e. style, education and certification) may play an important role in injury risk and prevention in various pediatric athlete populations. Other examples may include cross-training, sleep patterns, nutrition, and numerous additional psychosocial factors to those previously identified.

Evidence from descriptive epidemiological studies can be utilized in targeting relevant athlete groups [i.e. high-risk sports such as hockey, basketball, football, soccer (particularly indoor), and gymnastics], age groups (i.e. older adolescents) and skill levels (i.e. low-skill division in female adolescent soccer) in designing future research examining risk factors and prevention strategies in child and adolescent sport. Future studies examining prevention strategies such as preseason conditioning and proprioceptive balance training are warranted. Future RCTs examining optimal sport-specific injury prevention strategies should quantify and control for potential risk factors for injury in child and adolescent sport. It is critical to integrate basic science, laboratory and epidemiological research to maximize the understanding of mechanisms of injury, risk factors for injury, optimal prevention strategies, complete and appropriate treatment (i.e. medical, surgical and rehabilitation), and long-term effects of injury in youth sport. Long-term follow-up studies should be part of the future vision for research in injury prevention in youth sport. These will be critical, quantifying the long-term impact of pediatric sport injuries on future sport participation and the implications for the future health of our population (i.e. development of OA and other disease morbidity and mortality).

References

1   Lysens R, Steverlynck A, van den Auweele Y, Lefevre J, Renson R, Claessens A, et al: The predictability of sports injuries. Sports Med 1984;1:6–10.
2   Meeuwisse WH: Predictability of sports injuries: What is the epidemiological evidence? Sports Med 1991;12:8–15.
3   Canadian Fitness and Lifestyle Research Institute: http://www.cflri.ca/cflri/resources/pub.php#98pamrep. 2003.
4   Statistics Canada. Culture and Tourism Division: Canada's culture and heritage and identity: A statistical perspective. Ottawa, Ministry of Industry, 1997.
5   Backx FJG, Beijer HJM, Bol E, Erich WBM: Injuries in high-risk persons and high-risk sports. A longitudinal study of 1818 school children. Am J Sports Med 1991;19:124–130.

6   Bijur PE, Trumble A, Harel Y, Overpeck MD, Jone D, Scheidt PC: Sports and recreation injuries in US children and adolescents. Arch Pediatr Adolesc Med 1995;149:1009–1016.

7   Grimmer KA: Young people's participation in sports and recreational activities, and associated injury. South Australia, University of South Australia and Sports Medicine Australia, 1999.

8   Grimmer KA, Jones D, Williams J: Prevalence of adolescent injury from recreational exercise: An Australian perspective. J Adolesc Health 2000;27:1–6.

9   Northern Sydney Area Health Services, New South Wales Youth Injury Report, 1997.

10   Blair SN: Physical activity, physical fitness and health. Res Q Exerc Sport 1993;64:365–376.

11   Blair SN, Kohl HW, Barlow CE: Changes in physical fitness and all-cause mortality: A prospective study of healthy and unhealthy men. JAMA 1995;273:1093–1098.

12   Jebb S, Moore M: Contribution of a sedentary lifestyle and inactivity to the etiology of overweight and obesity: Current evidence and research issues. Med Sci Sports Exerc 1999;31:S534–S541.

13   Paffenbarger RS, Kamput JB, Lee IM: Changes in physical fitness and other lifestyle patterns influence longevity. Med Sci Sports Exerc 1994;26:857–865.

14   Daniel DM, Stone ML, Dobson BE: Fate of the ACL injured patient. A prospective outcome study. Am J Sports Med 1994;22:632–644.

15   Drawer F, Fuller CW: Propensity for osteoarthritis and lower limb joint pain in retired professional soccer players. Br J Sports Med 2001;35:402–408.

16   Gillquist J, Messner K: Anterior cruciate ligament reconstruction and the long-term incidence of gonarthrosis. Sports Med 1999;27:143–156.

17   van Mechelen W: Sports injury surveillance. One size fits all? Sports Med 1997;24:164–168.

18   Bienefeld M, Pickett W, Carr PA: A descriptive study of childhood injuries in Kingston, Ontario, using data from computerized injury surveillance system. Chronic Dis Can 1996;17:21–27.

19   Emery C: Risk factors for injury in child and adolescent sport: A systematic review of the literature. Clin J Sport Med 2003;13:256–268.

20   King MA, Pickett W, King ALJ: Injury in Canadian youth: A secondary analysis of the 1993–94 health behaviour in school-aged children survey. Can J Public Health 1998;89:397–401.

21   Abernethy L, MacAuley D: Impact of school sports injury. Br J Sports Med 2003;37:354–355.

22   Mummery WK, Spence JC, Vincenten JA, Voaklander DC: A descriptive epidemiology of sport and recreation injuries in a population-based sample: Results from the Alberta Sport and Recreation Injury Survey. Can J Public Health 1998;89:53–56.

23   Backx FJG, Erich WBM, Kemper ABA, Verbeek ALM: Sports injuries in school-aged children. An epidemiologic study. Am J Sports Med 1989;17:234–240.

24   McLain LG, Reynolds S: Sports injuries in a high school. Pediatrics 1989;84:446–450.

25   Messina DF, Farney WC, DeLee JC: The incidence of injury in Texas high school basketball. A prospective study among male and female athletes. Am J Sports Med 1999;27:294–299.

26   Roberts WO, Brust JD, Leonard BO: Youth ice hockey tournament injuries: Rates and patterns compared to season play. Med Sci Sports Exerc 1999;31:46–51.

27   Brust JD, Leonard BJ, Pheley A, Roberts WO: Children's ice hockey injuries. Am J Dis Child 1992;146:741–747.

28   Goldberg B, Rosenthal PP, Robertson LS, Nicholas JA: Injuries in youth football. Pediatrics 1988;81:255–261.

29   Zaricznyj B, Shattuck LJM, Mast TA, Robertson RV, D'Elia G: Sports-related injuries in school aged children. Am J Sports Med 1980;8:318–324.

30   Gallagher S, Finison K, Guyer B, Goodenough S: The incidence of injuries among 87,000 Massachusetts children and adolescents: Results of the 1980–81 statewide childhood injury prevention program surveillance system. Am J Public Health 1984;74:1340–1347.

31   Sorensen L, Larsen S, Rock N: The epidemiology of sports injuries in school aged children. Scand J Med Sci Sports 1996;6:281–286.

32   Stanitski CL, DeLee JC, Drez D (eds): Pediatric and Adolescent Sports Medicine. Philadelphia, WB Saunders Co, 1994

33   Caine DJ, Caine CG, Lindner KJ: Epidemiology of Sports Injuries. Illinois, Human Kinetics, 1996.

34   Emery CA: Does decreased muscle strength cause acute muscle strain injury in sport? A systematic review of the evidence. Phys Ther Rev 1999;4:79–85.

35   Emery CA, Meeuwisse WH: Risk factors for groin and abdominal strain injury in the National Hockey League Preseason: A multivariate approach. Med Sci Sports Exerc 1999;9:1423–1433.

36   Jones BH, Bovee MW, Harris JM, Cowan DN: Intrinsic risk factors for exercise-related injuries among male and female army trainees. Am J Sports Med 1993;21:705–710.

37   Pinto M, Kuhn JE, Greenfield MLV, Hawkins RJ: Prospective analysis of ice hockey injuries at the Junior A level over the course of a season. Clin J Sport Med 1999;9:70–74.

38   Tropp H, Ekstrand J, Gillquist J: Stabilometry in functional instability of the ankle and its value in predicting injury. Med Sci Sports Exerc 1984;16:64–66.

39   Tropp H, Ekstrand J, Gillquist J: Factors affecting stabilometry recordings of single leg stance. Am J Sports Med 1984;12:185–188.

40   Cahill BR, Griffith EH: Effect of preseason conditioning on the incidence and severity of high school football knee injuries. Am J Sports Med 1978;6:180–184.

41   de Loes M: Epidemiology of sports injuries in the Swiss organization 'Youth and Sports' 1987–1989. Injuries, exposure and risks of main diagnoses. Int J Sports Med 1995;16:134–138.

42   Garrick JG, Requa RK: Role of external support in the prevention of ankle sprains. Med Sci Sports 1973;5:200–203.

43   Lenaway DD, Ambler AG, Beaudoin DE: The epidemiology of school-related injuries: New perspectives. Am J Prev Med 1992;8:193–198.

44   Backous DD, Friedl KE, Smith NJ, Parr TJ, Carpine WD: Soccer injuries and their relation to physical maturity. Am J Dis Child 1988;142:839–842.

45   Graham CJ, Cleveland E: Left-handedness as an injury risk factor in adolescents. J Adolesc Health 1995;16:50–52.

46   Caine D, Knutzen K, Howe W, Keeler L, Sheppard L, Henrichs D, et al: A three-year epidemiological study of injuries affecting young female gymnasts. Phys Ther Sport 2003;4:10–23.

47   Caine D, Cochrane B, Caine C, Zemper E: An epidemiological investigation of injuries affecting young competitive female gymnasts. Am J Sports Med 1989;17:811–820.

48   Robey JM, Blyth CS, Mueller FO: Athletic injuries: Application of epidemiologic methods. JAMA 1971;217:184–189.

49   Mueller FO, Blyth CS: Fatalities from head and cervical spine injuries occurring in tackle football: 40 years experience. Clin Sports Med 1987;6:185–196.

50   Machold W, Kwasny O, Gassler P, et al: Risk of injury through snowboarding. J Trauma 2000;48:1109–1114.

51   Schmidt-Olsen S, Bunemann L, Lade V, Brassoe J: Soccer injuries of youth. Br J Sports Med 1985;19:151–154.

52   Pasque CL, Hewett TE: A prospective study of high school wrestling injuries. Am J Sports Med 2000;28:509–515.

53   Heidt RS, Sweeterman LM, Carlonas RL, Traub JA, Tekulve FX: Avoidance of soccer injuries with preseason conditioning. Am J Sports Med 2000;28:659–662.

54   Lyman S, Fleisig GS, Waterbor JW, Funkhouser EM, Pulley L, Andrews JR, et al: Longitudinal study of elbow and shoulder pain in youth baseball pitchers. Med Sci Sports Exerc 2001;33:1803–1810.

55   McMahon KA, Nolan T, Bennett CM, Carlin JB: Australian rules football injuries in children and adolescents. Med J Aust 1993;159:301–306.

56   Steele VA, White JA: Injury prediction in female gymnasts. Br J Sports Med 1986;20:31–33.

57   Sullivan JA, Gross RH, Grana WA, Garcia-Moral CA: Evaluation of injuries in youth soccer. Am J Sports Med 1980;8:325–327.

58   Wright KJ, De Cree C: The influence of somatotype, strength and flexibility on injury occurrence among female competitive Olympic style gymnasts – A pilot study. J Phys Ther Sci 1998;10:87–92.

59   Yde J, Nielsen AB: Sports injuries in adolescents' ball games: Soccer, handball and basketball. Br J Sports Med 1990;24:51–54.

60   Hoff G, Martin T: Outdoor and indoor soccer: Injuries among youth players. Am J Sports Med 1986;14:231–233.

61   Kaplan TA, Digel SL, Scavo VA, Arellana SB: Effect of obesity on injury risk in high school football players. Clin J Sport Med 1995;5:43–47.

62 Stuart MJ, Morrey MA, Smith AM, Meis JK, Ortiguera CJ: Injuries in youth football: A prospective observational cohort analysis among players aged 9–13 years. Mayo Clin Proc 2002;77: 317–322.

63 Lindner KJ, Caine D: Physical and performance characteristics of injured and injury-free female gymnasts. J Hum Mov Stud 1993;25:69–83.

64 Armstrong N, van Mechelen W (eds): Paediatric Exercise Science and Medicine. New York, Oxford University Press, 2000.

65 Bailey DA, Wedge JH, McCulloch RG, Martin AD, Bernhardson SC: Epidemiology of fractures of the distal end of the radius in children as associated with growth. J Bone Joint Surg 1989; 71A:1225–1231.

66 Bixler B, Jones RL: High school football injuries: Effects of a post-halftime warm-up and stretching routine. Fam Pract Res J 1992;12:131–139.

67 Grace TG, Sweetser ER, Nelson MA, Ydens LR, Skipper BJ: Isokinetic muscle imbalance and knee-joint injuries. J Bone Joint Surg 1984;66A:734–740.

68 Grana WA, Rashkin A: Pitcher's elbow in adolescence. Am J Sports Med 1980;8:333–336.

69 Grubbs N, Nelson RT, Bandy WD: Predictive validity of an injury score among high school basketball players. Med Sci Sports Exerc 1997;29:1279–1285.

70 Maffulli N, King JB, Helms P: Training in elite young athletes (the Training of Young Athletes (TOYA) Study): Injuries, flexibility and isometric strength. Br J Sports Med 1994;28:123–136.

71 Smith AD, Stroud L, McQueen C: Flexibility and anterior knee pain in adolescent elite figure skaters. J Pediatr Orthop 1991;11:77–82.

72 Woodford-Rogers B, Cyphert L, Denegar CR: Risk factors for anterior cruciate ligament injury in high school and college athletes. J Athl Train 1994;29:343–346,376–377.

73 Gleim GW, McHugh MP: Flexibility and its effects on sports injury and performance. Sports Med 1997;24:289–299.

74 Albright JA, Jokl P, Shaw R, Albright JP: Clinical study of baseball pitchers: Correlation of injury to the throwing arm and method of delivery. Am J Sports Med 1978;6:15–21.

75 Faelker T, Pickett W, Brison RJ: Socioeconomic differences in childhood injury: A population based epidemiologic study in Ontario, Canada. Inj Prev 2000;6:203–208.

76 Kerr GA, Minden H: Psychological factors related to the occurrence of athletic injuries. J Sport Exerc Psychol 1988;10:167–173.

77 Kolt G, Kirby R: Injury in Australian competitive gymnastics: A psychological perspective. Aust J Physiother 1996;42:121–126.

78 Smith AM, Stuart MJ, Wiese-Bjornstal DM, Gunnon C: Predictors of injury in ice hockey players: A multivariate, multidisciplinary approach. Am J Sports Med 1997;25:500–507.

79 Smith RE, Smoll FL, Ptacek JT: Conjunctive moderator variables in vulnerability and resiliency research: Life stress, social support and coping skills, and adolescent sport. J Pers Soc Psychol 1990;58:360–370.

80 Upton PAH, Roux CE, Noakes TD: Inadequate pre-season preparation of school-boy rugby players – A survey of players at 25 Cape Province high schools. S Afri Med J 1996;86:531–533.

81 Junge A, Rosch D, Peterson L: Prevention of soccer injuries: A prospective intervention study in youth amateur players. Am J Sports Med 2002;30:652–659.

82 Wedderkopp M, Kaltoft M, Lundgaard B, Rosendahl M, Froberg K: Prevention of injuries in young female players in European team handball. A prospective intervention study. Scand J Med Sci Sports 1999;9:41–47.

83 Bahr R, Lian O: A two-fold reduction in the incidence of acute ankle sprains in volleyball. Scand J Med Sci Sports 1997;7:172–177.

84 Caraffa A, Cerulli G, Projetti M, Aisa G, Rizzo A: Prevention of anterior cruciate ligament injuries in soccer. A prospective controlled study of proprioceptive training. Knee Surg Sports Traumatol Arthrosc 1996;4:19–21.

85 Hewett TE, Lindenfeld TN, Riccobene JV, Noyes FR: The effect of neuromuscular training on the incidence of knee injury in female athletes. Am J Sports Med 1999;27:699–705.

86 Myklebust G, Engebretsen L, Braekken IH, Skjolberg A, Olsen O, Bahr R: Prevention of ACL injuries in female handball players: A prospective intervention study over 3 seasons. Clin J Sports Med 2003;13:71–78.

87 Emery C, Cassidy D, Klassen T, Rosychuk R, Rowe B: The effectiveness of a proprioceptive balance-training program in healthy adolescents: A cluster randomized controlled trial (abstract). Am J Epidemiol 2004;159:S46.

88 Wedderkopp M, Kaltoft M, Holm R, Froberg K: Comparison of two intervention programmes in young female players in European handball – With and without ankle disc. Scand J Med Sci Sports 2003;13:371–375.

89 Marshall S, Mueller F, Kirby D, Yang J: Evaluation of safety balls and faceguards for prevention of injuries in youth baseball. JAMA 2003;289:568–574.

90 Emery CA, Meeuwisse WH: Risk factors for groin injuries in hockey. Med Sci Sports Exerc 2001;33:1423–1433.

91 MacKay M, Scanlan A, Olsen L: Sports and recreational injury prevention strategies: Systematic Review and Best Practices: Executive Summary. Vancouver, BC, BC Injury Research and Prevention Unit, 2001.

92 Janda DH, Maguire R, Mackesy D: Sliding injuries in college and professional baseball – A prospective study comparing standard and break-away bases. Clin J Sport Med 1999;3:78–81.

93 Sendre RA, Keating TM, Hornak JE, Newitt PA: Use of the Hollywood Impact Base and standard stationary base to reduce sliding and base-running injuries in baseball and softball. Am J Sports Med 1994;22:450–453.

94 Sitler M, Ryan J, Wheeler B: The efficacy of a semi-rigid ankle stabilizer to reduce acute ankle injuries in basketball: a randomized clinical study at Westpoint. Am J Sports Med 1994;22: 454–461.

95 Benson BW, Rose MS, Meeuwisse WH: The impact of face shield use on concussions in ice hockey: A multivariate analysis. Br J Sports Med 2002;36(1):27–32.

96 Benson BW, Mohtadi NG, Rose MS, Meeuwisse WH: Head and neck injury among intercollegiate ice hockey players wearing full versus half face shields. JAMA 1999;282:2328–2332.

97 Meeuwisse WH: Full facial protection reduces injuries in elite young hockey players. Clin J Sport Med 2002;12:406.

98 Pashby T: Eye injuries in Canadian amateur hockey. Can J Ophthalmol 1985;20:2–4.

99 Torg JS, Vegso JJ, Sennett B: The National Football Head and Neck Injury Registry: 14 year report on cervical quadriplegia (1971–1984). Clin Sports Med 1987;6:61–72.

100 Roberts WO, Brust JD, Leonard B, Hebert BJ: Fair-play rules and injury reduction in ice hockey. Arch Pediatr Adolesc Med 1996;150:140–145.

101 Watson RC, Singer CD, Sproule JR: Checking from behind in ice hockey: A study of injury and penalty data in the Ontario University Athletic Association hockey league. Clin J Sport Med 1996;6:111.

102 Tropp H, Askling C, Gillquist J: Prevention of ankle sprains. Am J Sports Med 1985;13:259–262.

103 Hoffman M, Payne VG: The effects of proprioceptive ankle disk training on healthy subjects. J Orthop Sports Phys Ther 1995;21:90–94.

104 Holme E, Magnusson SP, Becher K, Bieler T, Aagaard P, Kjaer M: The effect of supervised rehabilitation on strength, postural sway, position sense and re-injury risk after acute ankle ligament sprain. Scand J Med Sci Sports 1999;9:104–109.

105 Emery CA, Cassidy D, Klassen T, Rosychuk R: The effectiveness of a proprioceptive balance training program in healthy adolescents. 6th World Conference on Injury Prevention and Control (abstracts), Montreal, Quebec, 2002.

106 Macnab A, Smith T, Gagnon F, Macnab M: Effect of helmet wear on the incidence of head/face and cervical spine injuries in young skiers and snowboarders. Inj Prev 2002;8:324–327.

107 Thompson D, Rivara F, Thompson RS: Effectiveness of bicycle safety helmets in preventing head injuries: A case-control study. JAMA 1996;276:1968–1973.

108 Wingfield K, Matheson GO, Meeuwisse WH: Preparticipation evaluation: An evidence-based review. Clin J Sport Med 2004;14:109–122.

109 Tursz A, Crost M: Sports related injuries in children. A study of their characteristics, frequency, and severity, with comparison to other types of accidental injury. Am J Sports Med 1986;14: 294–299.

110 Wright IC, Neptune RR, van den Bogert AJ, Nigg BM: The effects of ankle compliance and flexibility on ankle sprains. Med Sci Sports Exerc 2000;31:260–265.

111 Thompson N, Halpern B, Curl W, Andrews J, Hunter S, McLeod W: High school football injuries: Evaluation. Am J Sports Med 1987;15:S97–S104.
112 Donner A, Klar N: Design and Analysis of Cluster Randomization Trials in Health Research. New York, Oxford University Press, 2000.
113 Rothman K, Greenland S: Modern Epidemiology, ed 2. Philadelphia, Lippincott-Raven Publishers, 1998.

Prof. C. A. Emery
Sport Medicine Centre, Faculty of Kinesiology
University of Calgary
2500 University Drive N.W.
Calgary, Alta., T2N 1N4 (Canada)
Tel. +1 403 220 4608, Fax +1 403 220 9489, E-Mail caemery@ucalgary.ca

Subject Index